D0624935

15-MINUTE YOGA

HEALTH, WELL-BEING, AND HAPPINESS THROUGH DAILY PRACTICE

ULRICA NORBERG

15-MINUTE YOGA
HEALTH, WELL-BEING, AND HAPPINESS THROUGH DAILY PRACTICE

PHOTOGRAPHY: ANDREAS LUNDBERG
TRANSLATED BY DIANA KATARZYNA BIEDNY

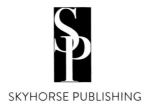

SKYHORSE PUBLISHING

Skyhorse Publishing books may be purchased in bulk at special discounts for sales promotion, corporate gifts, fund-raising, or educational purposes. Special editions can also be created to specifications. For details, contact the Special Sales Department, Skyhorse Publishing, 307 West 36th Street, 11th Floor, New York, NY 10018 or info@skyhorsepublishing.com.

Skyhorse® and Skyhorse Publishing® are registered trademarks of Skyhorse Publishing, Inc.®, a Delaware corporation.

www.skyhorsepublishing.com

10 9 8 7 6 5 4 3 2 1

Library of Congress Cataloging-in-Publication Data is available on file.

Cover design by Owen Corrigan

Print ISBN: 978-1-62914-517-4
Ebook ISBN: 978-1-62914-843-4

Printed in China

Contents

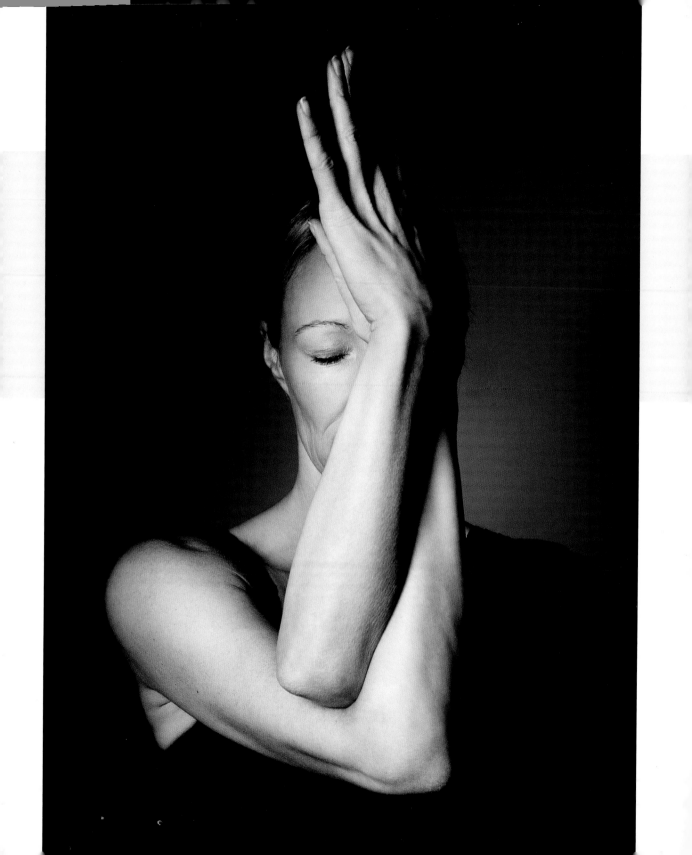

A Path to Well-being

"The intelligence behind the human being as a creation goes beyond our reason.
We can get an idea of this greatness only when we connect to the intelligence inside ourselves,
and our spirit through reflection and meditation."

YOGIRAJ ALAN FINGER

An individual's path to better health is generally different from that of another. We are all unique and the secret of success in yoga and other types of mind-body practice is to create a balancing practice for the body and mind. A mind body routine that strengthens and enlivens the body, quiets the mind, and gives life to the spirit. By practicing yoga, one can over time develop a self- balancing daily session that works toward what we need rather than giving in to what the mind wants.

For me, yoga has been an invaluable tool to create better balance in my my everyday life, in my work, and in my relationship with myself and the people around me. Yoga's focus on the interaction between the inner and outer aspects of everything, and how to merge them together, is the essence of why I and many others feel this way.

One of yoga's many gifts to humanity is the techniques and methods which have been tested, reflected upon, and ennobled over millennia. Some of these techniques are simple but effective, and through a regular exercise they help us to move more gracefully into better balance mentally, physically, and spiritually. Ancient yoga texts place particular emphasis on the importance of step-by-step equanimity in the practice, in order to not overwhelm the senses or the body, and to train the brain and heart to connect and be more stable, in every way. In many techniques, one sense is used in order to strengthen another, through one side of the body to balance the other, to go from doing to being, inner focus to outer focus, and so on. And through rest, we can find activity and vice versa. The word "health" derives from the Old English word *hælth*, which originally meant whole. Yoga is a way to become whole by integrating opposites—what we have within us interacts with what is outside of us. Then we reflect upon that merge and meditate before action.

We humans have an incredible capacity within us. And yoga helps us to understand our potential and through that to live a fuller life. Through a regular yoga practice, you can learn how to control the blood flow in your brain in order to strengthen the centers that control various mental and physical functions.

First we align the body with the help of breathing properly, and then through visualization and concentration exercises, we try to direct our attention to specific locations in the body to thereby recover the power of the brain and strengthen different body parts.

In this book, I focus on three aspects of yoga practice: breath, energy, and the physical body, as well as how to enhance the interaction between them and how they can be combined through short but effective yoga sessions—15 minutes a day.

The suggested practice sequences I have put together, which you can find in the back of the book, are all designed so that you start to work on merging the opposites I have mentioned: activity with recovery, more body in one, more mind in one, balance both right and left hemispheres and both sides of the body as well as building and recovering exercises. I have mixed yin yoga, which focuses on targeting the connective tissue with an aim of creating better circulation, more elasticity, and a harmonious mind, with yang yoga—energizing exercises to strengthen the muscle tissue. The mix of activity and rest creates power and stability in equal doses on the inside and on the outside. This way of practicing yoga has helped me a lot in my work and life in general. I hope you will appreciate how the programs are varied, and that they will do you good. Use them according to your own needs, circumstances, and goals, and then it will hopefully feel invigorating and motivating.

I wish you all the best.
Namaste,

Ulrica

THE YIN AND YANG YOGA

Physical yoga, called hatha yoga, works consistently with the balance of opposites in the practice, activity (*ha* in Sanskrit) and recovery (*tha*), in a way where one synchronizes the exercises that works the muscle tissue (*ha*) as much as the connective tissue (*tha*) in order to balance the force within an individual, *prana*. The *ha* and *tha* definitions come from the Indian tradition of yoga, while similar interactions of opposites in Chinese Taoism are called yin and yang. The concepts of yin and yang are often better recognized in the west, which is why modern yoga often borrows them to describe the relationship between opposites.

Yin yoga exercises are characterized by holding the poses longer and in stillness, in order to release tension, free locked-up *prana* (life force), and mobility, while yang yoga targets the muscle tissue and involves movement in flow with the breath, creating strength and stability.

The purpose of yin yoga is to create a greater elasticity in the connective tissue. The circulation in the muscles is promoted and yin yoga also makes it easier to release tensions and mental stress. In this book you will find a number of beneficial yin exercises that you are welcome to try.

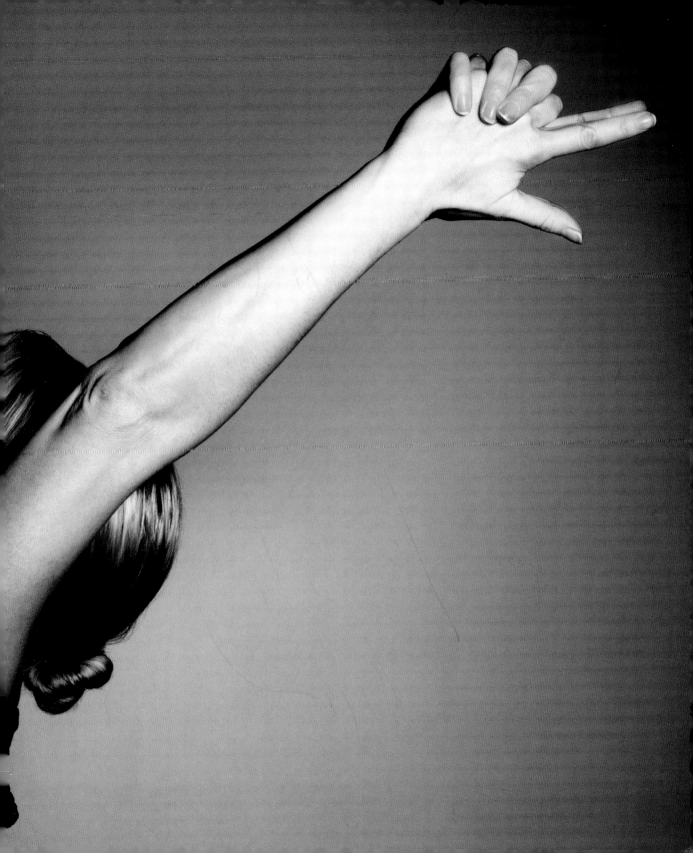

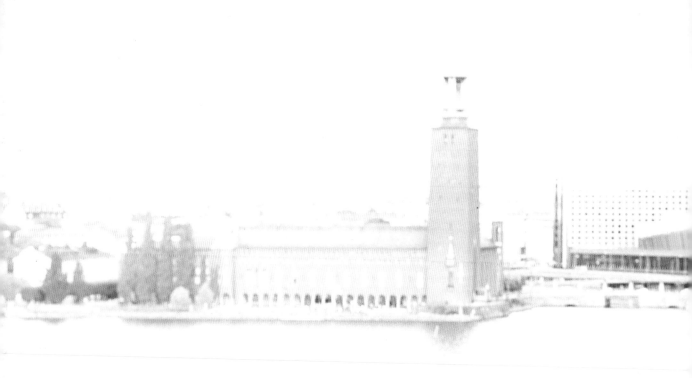

BASIC YOGA TERMS
What you often hear us yoga teachers talk about when we teach:

Alignment
Posture Technique. There is great emphasis on how different body parts are corrected into poses, *asana*, so that the yoga exercise will be ergonomic and provide stability in the joints.

Prana
Means life-force in Sanskrit. When you experience good circulation in a certain part of the body, or calmness after you have done a yoga exercise, you have given room for more life-giving force to flow in there. Yogis consider *prana* to be a tremendous healing power that we all have within us. It's just about releasing it, and through yoga, prohibiting it from being locked in any way.

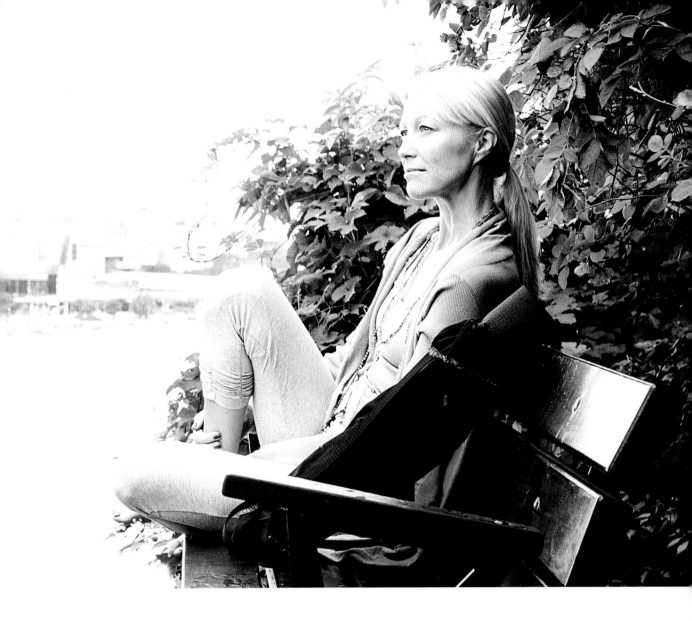

"BY TAKING ONE STEP AT A TIME THE IMPOSSIBLE BECOMES POSSIBLE."

T.K.V. DESIKACHAR

CHAPTER 1

Why Yoga?

Yoga means "bring together" or "to join" in Sanskrit, the ancient Indian language. It involves the reconciliation of different sorts of polarities in order to find balance and stability between them. Yoga refers to all contra-positions involving the body (in yoga we work to bring together front and back, outside and inside, upward and downward, contraction and extent), or what we experience with our senses (to be still and in motion, to listen and speak, to look and to close our eyes, to feel and express). It can also involve the balance between daily rhythms and shifts (night and day), or how different situations are perceived (enticing and challenging) and so on.

The body and mind constitute the foundation of our reality as we understand it, and these two aspects are expressions of the contradictions inherent in life: that which we can touch and visibly affect, and that which we cannot touch or see, yet can perceive and also affect with the mind—behaviors, ways of relating, and the ability to focus. Aspects which appear to be opposites always exist in relationship to each other. Yoga develops, unites, and balances opposites by allowing the body to meet the mind through the breath that unites them, in the moment, in the now.

For many people starting yoga, the first approach is through the physical aspects of yoga—*asana* (postures). When one starts practicing yoga it is usually in order to reduce stress, get in shape, or strengthen the mind. When one attends a yoga class, one is encouraged to initially draw most of the attention on the actual shape of the poses (posture). As the body learns, responds to, and adapts to the techniques, the practice becomes more stable, whilst one learns better posture, resulting in a more exiting and pleasurable process.

Gradually one usually becomes more interested in breathing techniques, mind practice, meditation, and yoga's deeper technical aspects, and then the effect of the yoga practice becomes more noticeable, not only in the connective tissue and the nervous system, but also in the way we move through life more gracefully. This is due to an increased oxygenation of the body and as well as reduced stress and tension. Paying attention to the vicissitudes of breathing, noticing changes and the different sensations that come and go in the body, as well as being able to record thoughts and feelings, are all equally important parts of yoga exercise. Forging a link between the body, mind, and spirit provides many other health benefits. In addition to that, you become stronger, healthier, and more agile.

Over time and after several encounters with your body and mind through yoga practice, when the physical health and the mind become stable, many yoga students develop an interest for what lies beneath the physical aspects—that which is not visible but rather experienced and cannot be put into words—awareness. The developmental process, which starts when one begins to practice yoga, usually occurs in three steps. First you reach the physical and mental process, then you move into the psychic or emotional process, and finally the symbolic or integrating process where one reaches better balance overall. All is one. And one is all. This is the purpose of yoga.

The Physical and Mental Process

When we start with yoga it affects us mostly on the physical and mental plane. Perhaps this was also the intention when we got on the mat for the first time. We know the effect of the practice when we become aware of our physical limitations, get sore, experience how difficult it can be to coordinate breathing, movement, and concentration inwards, and find that it is a challenge to attain the inner focus that allows us to concentrate on one thing during a longer period of time. Many reach insight on what an extraordinary power breathing is—something many take for granted, have never thought of or been aware of before.

When I started practicing yoga, I found it boring at times because I thought there was not enough action and movement in the practice. But afterwards, I felt so good that it led me to continue. I remember the first time I was sufficiently stable in a position, and I really felt a great difference when I was able to breathe like the teacher told me to. I felt strong and relaxed at the same time. It was such a cool feeling. Many yogis stay in this developmental phase for a long time. But gradually, many tend to explore further into philosophies, positions, and techniques. They will discover new tools in how to enhance physical, mental, and spiritual health.

The Psychic/Emotional Process

After a period of practice, you start to become familiar with the flow of the practice and the respective poses are recognized. The breathing is well integrated and you can notice the difference in the practice when you breathe properly and can easily focus your gaze, *drishti* in Sanskrit, in poses and meditation. You come to a point in your development where you do yoga regularly and it does not require as much energy to control the body. You get into the poses automatically and you are well aware of many techniques.

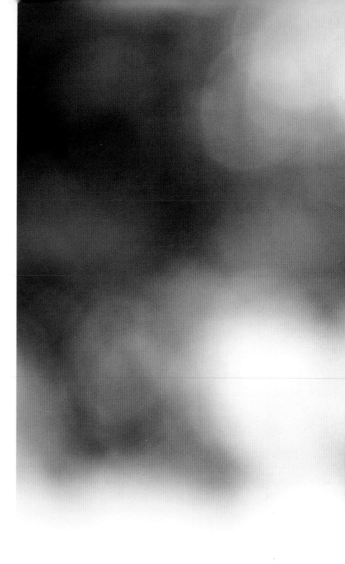

This is when you are beginning to reconcile your mind and your body, and you have a greater presence and a deeper focus. The flow of the practice will allow you to work even more on your concentration, so you can shut out all distractions and go into yourself, be able to listen to your breathing, notice the changes and nuances in the experience of a yoga pose, and thus tailor it to your own needs.

Outside of the mat, you bring the lessons from the practice with you into your life. You may not be as quick on reacting outwardly, but your progress is shown in that you are more accepting of your surroundings, and better able to mark your own limits more humbly. You begin to understand what makes you feel good in life and how you want to live.

The Symbolic/Integrative Process

When you reach this phase, yoga is a natural part of your everyday life. Your yoga gives you a perspective on life and you are more likely to reflect more and not be so quick to judge. You are now experiencing the effects of yoga. All along, you make choices according to need and in accordance with your search for balance, and not by ambition and perfection.

You look at life from a more balanced perspective and you start to realize that yoga is not just about the physical practice poses, *asanas* in Sanskrit, but that they, as well as everything else belonging to yoga, is a path leading you to understand who you are and what makes you feel good.

Essentially, practicing yoga is about a refinement in the ability to be alert and have presence in all of life's situations and events. Yoga aims to develop greater self-knowledge and consciousness, which in turn leads to having greater self-awareness and being able to respect and integrate with your surroundings and the world around you without losing your grip.

YOGA, A RELIGION?

Yoga is not a religion. It does not have the spiritual dogma and doctrines that most religious traditions have. Yoga relies on individual discoveries and personal inquiry, whereas religion has a collective moral thought. Yoga has always been about developing an individual reflection in order to bring life's opposites together to help a person become spiritually free and strong in him or herself. That inner balance then reflects upon the society positively. When one has inner peace, it brings outer peace.

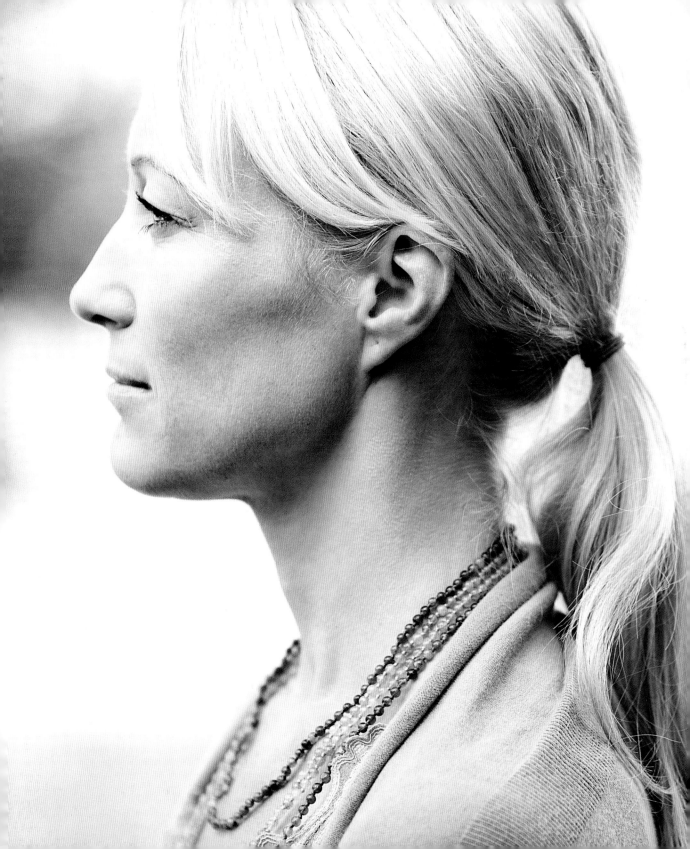

"Body without breath has no value, and if we have a body and breath but if there is no thinking, then that human being is also of no use. And if there is a human being who thinks, who breathes and whose body functions, that is also meaningless if he does not direct all his energies, mind, action and speech according to the purpose of life."

SWAMI RAMA

CHAPTER 2

Breathing

A bodily system that carries a central and strategic impact on the flow of energy in the body and mind, the respiratory system—the breath. Breathing provides the body with oxygen which is the body's fuel. The rhythm, direction, and depth of breathing affect the body's energy balance. With each breath, oxygen and energy flows through the body in waves, electromagnetic impulses controlled by the nervous system and the brain. The flow of energy creates and supports the tissues of the body, and if the energy field changes highly enough, it also changes the physical body.

Breathing is the only physical process that can be both voluntary and involuntary. You can breathe consciously, breathe as you wish, or ignore it and then the body simply breathes on its own. The body cannot function without breathing, so if conscious control of breathing is abandoned, the unconscious reflex takes over and respiration proceeds automatically.

Breathing affects the nervous system. When you inhale, the sympathetic nervous system is affected, and the body activates. When you exhale, the parasympathetic nervous system, the recovering part, is affected, leading to a relaxation of the body. So by taking full breaths—inhaling and exhaling—the body experiences both activity and relaxation in one breathing cycle, which balances the nervous system.

A well-balanced breath not only strengthens our overall health, but also prepares us to better deal with chaos, trauma, and challenging situations. Not by denial, embellishment or alteration, but just by becoming more present in the moment and more aware without becoming too emotionally involved. Sometimes you have to know when to be in control and when to let go of it. Overtime, your yoga practice helps to give you the balance you need to create greater clarity on when one or the other is justified.

THE FOUR ASPECTS OF BREATH

1. *Pooraka, inhalation.*
2. *Rechaka, exhalation.*
3. *Antar kumbhaka, holding the breath after inhalation— breathing-pause with oxygen in the lungs. Activating— increases the energy in the body.*
4. *Bahir kumbhaka, holding the breath after exhalation—breathing-pause with carbon dioxide in the lungs. Calming—softening the energy in the body.*

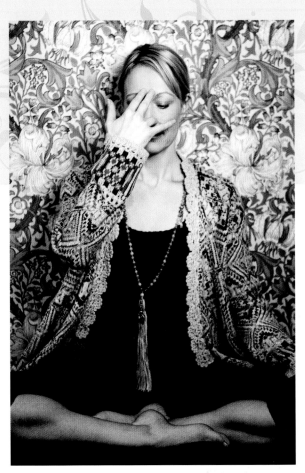

Yoga Strengthens the Respiratory Muscles

Each breath consists of two activities: inhalation and exhalation. The inhalation is a controlled muscular effort conducted by three distinct sets of muscle groups: those working between the ribs, toward the ribs, and then the diaphragm which is the "floor" in the chest (thorax).

Our exhalation is performed by means of the transversal abdominal muscles, the transversus abdominis, and the pelvic floor.

When breathing is proper, a sort of an internal massage occurs in the organs of the abdomen. On inhalation the diaphragm moves downward, becomes flatter, and massages the liver as the blood is lead to the organ, in order to consequently be forced out by means of exhalation to give pressure to the heart. When we exhale, the transverse abdominal muscles, the muscles between the ribs, and the intercostal muscles activate and the withheld air that

otherwise would remain in the lungs is forced out.

Yoga-breathing is done through the nose, with the mouth closed, to retain the heat in the body and thus save energy. When you breathe in through your mouth, the body cools down and in yoga, we want to keep the heat inside.

ABOUT THE DIAPHRAGM

The diaphragm is a domed muscle plate that separates the chest from the abdominal cavity. If you look at it from below it looks like an open umbrella, and from above like a hill.

Breathing Exercises

Controlling the breathing so that it is long, deep, and even is one way to calm and strengthen the nervous system, and also a condition for stabilizing the mind. Balancing the mind is a prerequisite to tame the universal energy, *prana* or life force. The one who has learned to control *prana* has learned to master the body and mind.

In yoga this is called *pranayama,* also in Sanskrit, where *prana* means "life force" and *ayama* means "extension/control of the life force." According to yogic teachings, the relationship between breathing and mind is reciprocal. A particular state of mind results in a particular kind of breathing and vice versa, and when we consciously introduce a certain breathing technique, we can produce the corresponding state of mind. By consciously making breathing deep, even, and regular, we help the body to cleanse, release tensions, and increase the ability to relax.

Introduction to Yoga Breathing

When you learn proper breathing, it is good to take it one step at a time:

1. The first step is getting to know your own individual respiratory pattern. Conscious concentration on your own breathing makes your breathing rhythm calmed to a more relaxed and balanced flow. Sit in a comfortable position, such as cross-legged, or you can lie down. Close your eyes. Observe your existing respiratory pattern. Is your breath even or uneven? Does it feel hard or soft, and is breathing high or low in your chest? Try to gradually make the breathing deeper, more even, and calmer, focusing on the respiratory movement in the solar plexus, which is around the midriff.

2. The second step is to create a good body posture. Visualize a line running from the root of your spine to the top of your crown and thereby create an extension of the spine (to reduce an unnecessary load on the vertebras and disks, and to create a better circulation through the lumbar musculature). Continue the visualization and watch how the inhalation is "pulled up" from the front of the spine to the top of the crown, and how it "flows down" on the back of the spine while you exhale.

3. Finally, focus on the movement of your chest. Feel how the diaphragm and the chest expand during inhalation, outward/backward, and slowly sink toward the spine as you exhale. Concentrate on making your inhalation and exhalation equal in length. This

---

EFFECTS OF BREATHING EXERCISES IN YOGA

If you have never practiced pure breathing exercises, various symptoms may occur during or after performing the exercises. You may experience mild itching on your body, tickling on the skin, and you may feel heavy or light, cold or hot. These feelings are temporary and will disappear.

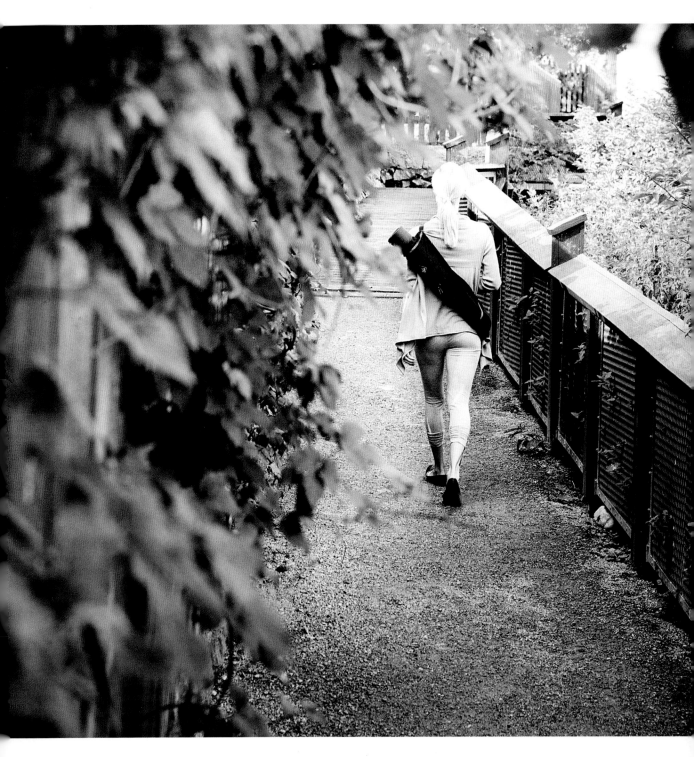

Ujjayi pranayama
Expanding breath

Sanskrit: *uj* = expand, *jayi* = gain, exaltation
Pronounced oo-jai

This breathing technique is mainly used while performing different yoga poses. *Ujjayi* is characterized by a subtle whispering sound that occurs in the throat when you breathe through your nose with your mouth closed. This technique is the opposite of your otherwise unconscious breathing, because you inhale and exhale actively and consciously. The characterizing feature of *ujjayi* is to work with this breathing sound silently to oneself. *Ujjayi* breath makes it easier to maintain focus and heat in the body as the circulation increases. Keep the breathing in the back of the throat to increase pressure in the trachea, thus creating more muscle work for the diaphragm. This breathing technique is an effective way to strengthen the diaphragm, increase circulation in the muscle area around the solar plexus, and help to increase focus on what you do.

1. PREPARATION

Sit or stand comfortably. Start by focusing on your exhalation. Exhale with your mouth closed, and concentrate on sinking the lower part of your chest downward and inward toward the spine. This means that all the air is pumped out from your lungs. Now try to hold your breath for a moment, then let go. You will notice how you automatically inhale again and how the thoracic lower part expands.

2. FINDING *UJJAYI*

Now try to take the breath one step further by creating an active exhalation and inhalation. Start by whispering an "ahhh" or "uuu" with your mouth open when you exhale. Feel the vibration in your throat. Then inhale and at the same time whisper "ahhh" or "uuu." Slowly fill your lungs with air. With the help of the sound, try to fill up and empty out your lungs of air. Now do the same thing but with your mouth closed. Your exhalation will now allow more wheezing.

3. BALANCING

Strive to create the same sound on inhalation as well as exhalation. If you start coughing or feeling sick while exercising *ujjayi* breathing, you have exerted yourself too much. Breaths should be smooth and long, and you should strive to keep your shoulders relaxed and have springiness in your chest. Do not forget to also try to expand the chest in the thoracic spine. Visualize yourself breathing into the back: 30 percent of breathing capacity is found there. *Ujjayi* combined with yoga poses provides complete tools for achieving endurance and strength, a better balance, and becoming more flexible and agile.

"Breathing is like a thin thread that can become strong and powerful and be an excellent tool to help us handle situations that otherwise could seem impossible. Breathing is the bridge between our physical and psychological self and the element that makes it possible for the body, soul, and mind to become one unity. Breathing is like an engine that makes us live but conscious breathing can also make us stronger, more resistant, healthier, calmer, and harmonic."

THICH NHAT HANH

Nadi shodhana

Alternate nostril breathing

Sanskrit: *nadi* = energy channel, *shodhana* = purification

Begin with *ujjayi* breathing but now through one nostril at a time. Sit in a comfortable seated position with a straight back and hands resting on the knees with the palms facing upward. Let the index finger and thumb meet on the left hand. Place the right index and middle fingertips in between your eyebrows and place your right thumb and ring finger over each side of the nostrils.

Keep your little finger straight and relaxed. From a beginner's level one always begins with inhalation through the left nostril and ends with expiration on the right side.

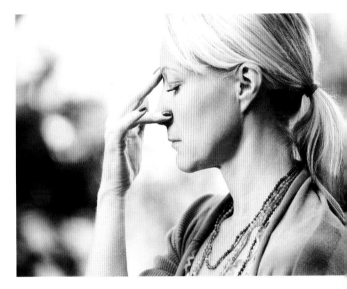

1. Exhale completely. Close your right nostril first with your right thumb.
2. Inhale slowly through your left nostril until you fill your lungs completely.
3. Close both nostrils with your ring finger and thumb.
4. Release your thumb and exhale slowly through your right nostril until you cannot exhale anymore (without force).
5. Close both nostrils.
6. Release your thumb and inhale through your right nostril.
7. Close both nostrils.
8. Release your ring finger and exhale through your left nostril.
9. This is one round. Repeat 4–6 more times.

RHYTHM IS in through left, close both, out through right, close both, in through right, close off, out through left, and so forth. Then, lie down on your back and rest for a minute or more.

Alternate nostril breathing, *nadi shodana*, contributes to increased focus, calmness, clarity of thought, and concentration, and is recommended to those who have mentally or intellectually demanding work. This technique increases the vitality of the nervous system and body organs, lowers stress levels and the feeling of anxiety in the body.

21

CHAPTER 3

Energy

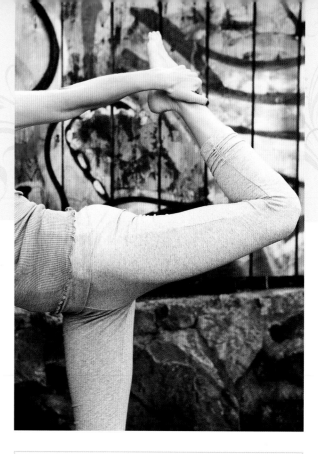

Energy can be described as something that causes change, as a force that sets something in motion. Energy may be stored or be slightly transformed in various forms. The word "energy" comes from the Greek word "energeia," which means activity or action. But it was not until the 1800s that the connection between heat and motion, the so-called energy principle, was discovered. In broad terms, the energy principle means that energy can neither be created nor destroyed, but converted between different forms: for example, between mechanical, electrical and chemical, and thermal energy.

The yoga philosophy has pointed out for millennia that us humans are driven by and made up of energy, and that yoga and meditation is all about getting to understand this and how we can use the energy within us in the best way. In yoga practice, we strive to influence the energy balance in the body, mind, and soul so that these three aspects can interact better for us to reach our ultimate potential as a human being. Fundamentally, energy balance is about where and on what to target and focus your energy. If you want to become stronger, you cannot just work with activity. You need to alternate it with rest. If you want to get better at communication, it is not enough just to communicate. You also need to rest from all communication.

In many yoga techniques you work through one sense to strengthen another, through one side of the body or brain to balance the other, and so on. We use rest to get active and vice versa.

WEST MEETS EAST

Neuroscientists have studied the brains of meditating Buddhist monks with MRI and discovered that meditation alters, redesigns, and repairs certain parts of the brain. This leads to feeling better both mentally and physically. This is interesting because scientists previously believed that after a certain age the brain could not develop anymore, but new research has led them to reconsider.

Modern brain research in the field of neuroplasticity, which explores the brain's ability to change and heal, is on the same track as the yoga masters. "Neuroplasticity" comes from two words, "neuron" (or nerve cell) and "plasticity," which means ability to reshape. This proves that the way in which we think, learn things, and act affects the physical structure and the functional organization of the brain.

The word "meditation" comes from the Latin "meditare" which means to contemplate, reflect upon, and keep in mind. Meditation has several dimensions. It could for example mean that you are thinking a lot and seriously about something, perhaps regarding a move, if you really should take that job, how to act in a certain matter, or what kind of education you should choose. These reflections can last for a long time. Even a movie or a book can touch you and leave you pensive. Meditation, from a yogic perspective, is not merely a technique that we add to ourselves in the same way that we learn a language, or gain knowledge of how a computer works. Here, it is rather about deep reflection.

Practicing yoga in the two different ways I suggest in this book—a combination of yin and yang, between passive activity and active flow—offers us favorable conditions to neutralize negative energy and create better circulation, power, and creativity in both body and mind, and in life in general. Then meditation ought to be added to make a strong and durable health state.

Meditation—A Path to Energy Balance

Meditation is a mind practice that includes several stages and dimensions of consciousness. What it all comes down to is going into a no-mind state of conciousness by concentrating on staying in the present, in the moment, with the help of an activity or a specific technique or method.

Meditation is an upgrade and rest for the mind so that it can function better in its active state. Meditation helps to disperse and calm down thoughts and feelings which are inextricably linked to your daily life. The mind processes memories, current problems, and plans for the future; all of this, in turn, evokes lots of emotions. Through meditation, you can objectively observe these emotions without drowning in them or identifying with them. This reduces the risk of suffering from unwelcome and harmful thoughts and feelings.

THE POWER OF MEDITATION

Meditation has the following positive effects:

- Increases the ability for deep relaxation
- Increases the capacity for controlled and conscious tension
- Improves the capacity of concentration and focus
- Improves breathing
- Reduces stress levels in the body
- Increases the feeling of quality-of-life
- Creates greater self-awareness and well-being
- Increases mental capacity
- Increases lung capacity
- Improves digestion

Meditation has shown to have the following clinical effects on the body:

- Helps to prevent joint problems (small but clear effects, improved functional ability)
- Can relieve pain on many levels
- Relieves headache
- Reduces high blood pressure (breathing lowers blood pressure)

MEDITATION TECHNIQUES

Focusing On an Object—*drishti*

Here, you focus on an object with your gaze. Choose an emotionally neutral object that speaks of the same thing you wish to accomplish in your meditation. If it is insight, perhaps choose a candle, or if it's grounding you seek, a beautiful stone is the way to go. Focusing your eyes on a lit candle or on the smoke rising from lit incense is a popular technique that works for many. You can also focus on a flower in a vase, a statue or figurine, or an object from nature. Use the technique with open or semi-closed eyes to create a gentler glance.

1. Sit comfortably on the floor or on a chair.
2. Place your object in front of you and focus your eyes on it.
3. Set an egg timer for 10 minutes or a time of your choice.
4. Gently fix your eyes on the object. Start studying it. Use your mind to observe its outline and try to see new aspects of the object. As soon as your thoughts take off elsewhere focus on the object again and look. Soon your eyes will close. Try and stay in that state with the help of your breath and by "seeing" your object as an image on the screen of the mind.
5. When the timer sounds, slowly open your eyes and fix your gaze on a fixed point in front of you. Take 4 deep breaths.
6. End by lying down on your back for 3–5 minutes, try to close your eyes, and take long deep breaths. In Sanskrit, this method is called *drishti* and means "point of view," "gaze," or "reflection." *Drishti* is also known as the gaze focus in the actual yoga practice.

Aware Focused Breathing—*apa japa*

Apa japa is classified both as a breathing technique as well as a meditation technique, and is designed to increase awareness on all levels in the yogi. It is based on focusing the mind on breathing until the mind begins to calm down and concentration arises. Strive to emulate the slow and regular breathing that you have while sleeping. When endorphins are released in the body, a sense of calm arises and the brain is provided with more oxygenated blood.

1. Sit comfortably on the floor or on a chair.
2. Set an egg timer for 10 minutes or a time of your choice.
3. Start listening to and observing your breathing pattern just as it is, without changing it; just follow it. Breathing is now your object of focus in meditation. Study every nuance in the breath as well as every feeling that arises and that the breath evokes—how it feels in the stomach and chest when you breathe, how it feels when the air flows in and out through your nose, the temperature, and so on. It is important not to start evaluating or analyzing the breathing but just listening to it. Try to resist becoming involved in what you are focusing on.
4. Breathing becomes calm and deep, thoughts are quieter and less attractive to follow, and your eyes close.
5. When the timer sounds, slowly open your eyes and fix your gaze on a fixed point in front of you. Take 4 deep breaths.
6. End by lying down on your back for 3–5 minutes, try to close your eyes, and take long deep breaths.

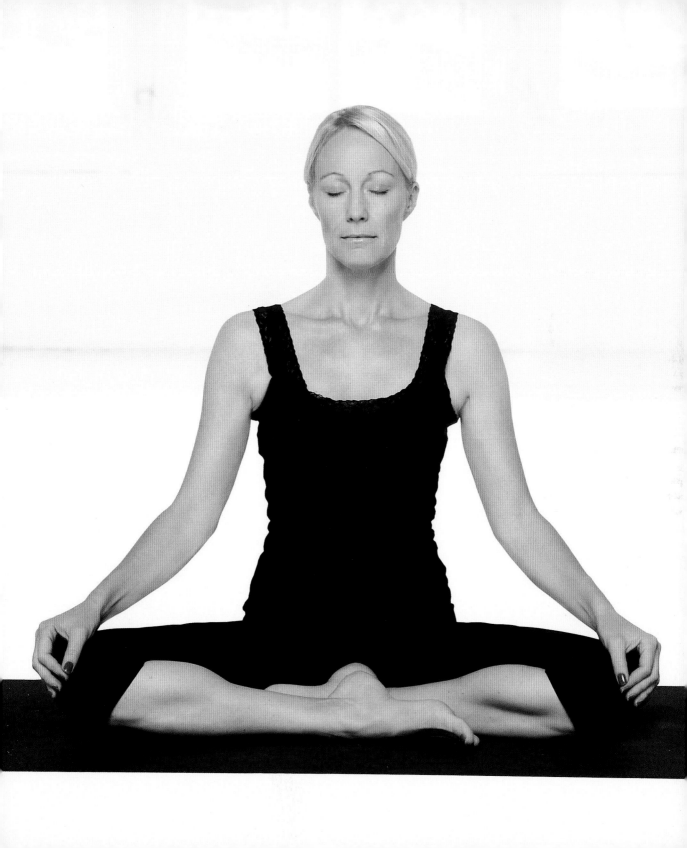

CHAPTER 4

The Physical Body

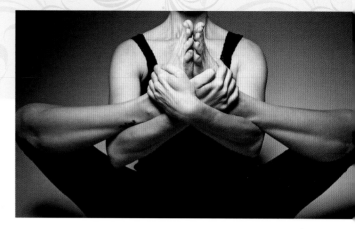

Sthiram Sukham Asanam

– Yoga Sütra, book 2, verse 46

"Yoga poses should be steady, comfortable, and instill a sense of lightness, freedom, and just enough challenge." This is what the quote above explains.

Another proverb from the yoga tradition is: "You only are as young as your spine is." In yoga, namely all poses originate from the spine. Our spine is designed to constantly strive for balance in order to cope with everything the body is exposed to.

This is important to remember, because when we have back problems or imbalances, we get irritated and annoyed because our back is not functioning well, and we often try to get rid of the pain with an overuse of medicine instead of rest or by strengthening it through exercise.

Breathing, Posture, and Support

In physical yoga we focus primarily on three things to make practice more effective and conscious, and to avoid injuries.

1. BREATHING

Enhance *prana* flowing freely. Taking full, even, and deep breaths in order to oxygenate the blood that circulates in the body as well as listening to your breathing to increase focus and presence.

2. POSTURE

Sitting, standing, and lying down in a good posture. Yoga uses the English term alignment to describe this. To strive for correct, individually balanced positioning in poses and in motion is more important than to be ruled by perfection in a pose.

3. SUPPORT

In our practice, we gather support and stability through where we put our gaze—*drishti*—and we activate the muscles in a specific area, such as the pelvic floor and abdomen for example. We achieve relaxation and increased circulation via tools such as blankets, blocks, and bolsters.

In yoga, the goal of all of body poses, the so-called asanas, is to strive for the feeling of stability and comfort (*sthira* in Sanskrit), as well as harmony, flow, and circulation (called *sukha* in Sanskrit) in the performance of the body poses.

If you feel resistance and the exercise feels mentally challenging, you should not push yourself any further.

Breathe, pause, stay, or modify the pose. It is very important to be cautious with the aforementioned, for the precise reason that we often want to hurry and rush forward as quickly as possible. If we listen too much to our mind and not our body, it is very likely that one day we will get hurt in practice. All asanas are related to each other in one way or another and have the mission to strengthen the muscles around the spine, known as postural muscles, which allow us to stand, sit, run, lie down, and so forth, in a more qualitative way.

The focus is on the hip flexor muscle, the pelvic floor, the abdominal and lumbar spine muscles, the thoracic muscles, and the thoracic spine muscles.

These are the muscle groups that hold up the spine and make us stable and agile. They are also much related to the quality of our breathing. If these muscles are weakened, problems with the back, hips, shoulders, blood circulation, digestion, and more will often arise. This is a common problem today, due largely to our lifestyle. We have unilateral movement patterns. Often we sit and lie too much and we are way too still. Moreover, we stress and make erroneous priorities in terms of our health. *Asana* in Sanskrit means "to sit," and the goal of yoga poses is to learn how to stand, walk, and sit with an anatomically balanced and implicitly good posture, and to be comfortable in our own skin. Therefore, the actual execution of the yoga pose is more important than the pose itself.

The Asanas will prepare you so that you can achieve mental and spiritual balance as well as control in everyday life, and thus have a "good posture" regardless of the situation. This is how the asanas have both an external and internal dimension. In other words, asanas lead us through both external and internal movements—the exterior in the form of body poses and movement sequences, and the interior in the form of breathing, focus, concentration, and mental clarity. This creates the necessary momentum to be able to find stability in body, soul, and mind.

BREATHING AND POSITION IN FOCUS

Breathing is what unifies our body with our awareness, and movement, combined with a proper breathing technique, is the basis of all physical yoga. When breathing becomes stronger and we manage to focus on it more, we increase our body awareness, improve our balance, and enhance our posture in the movements. And the experience in the yoga poses feels more natural, as in "doing it right."

In yoga, having a good posture is very important. It reduces harmful stress patterns and increases blood circulation around the joints. Posture involves bones, joints, and muscles. By focusing on our way of keeping our body when walking, sitting, and standing, many back and muscle problems can be avoided. A good body posture generally also gives a better charisma.

THE SPINE—THE BODY'S VERTICAL LINE

The cooperation between the back, bones, joints, and muscles allows us to stand upright, sit, walk, run, jump, and more. The spine is composed of four parts: the pelvis, the lumbar, the thoracic, and cervical spine (the neck). It is supported by large and small muscles, and ligaments that attach the vertebrae and the bones. The muscles hold up the body and help us to undertake major and minor movements.

We are all born with a different form of our spine, pelvis, and shoulders. Some are rounder in the upper back while others are straighter. The same goes for the lower back. Some have a significant arching in their back while others have almost none. Thus we inherit much of our posture from our ancestors, but what then affects our heritage is how we live our lives: exercise, fitness, work, and how we feel psychologically.

Today, more than 70 percent of the Western adult population suffers from some sort of back problems. It is often related to how we live our lives—how we move, or rather not move, how we think, eat, sleep, communicate, and feel. Everything plays a role in how our back feels. If our back feels good then we feel good, and vice versa.

Rehabilitation of back problems must of course be based on each individual in order to be effective. Despite this, it is still better to start exercising your back instead of being passive and just waiting for the health of our back to return. It does not happen automatically. The most important thing in all back rehabilitations is to perform the exercises with calmness and in a dialogue with the breathing, and by always listening to your body's reactions.

All asanas are based on and strengthen the musculature around the spine. In yoga, we speak of the quest to become "more centered," and this means that we try to strengthen the back and reduce imbalances. It also allows a stronger nervous system that improves the whole general condition.

In yoga, the spine is seen as a *merudanda,* a high mountain. When your back is in balance, you are in balance, and symbolically you then climb this mountain to get a better perspective on life and yourself. It creates self-distance, strength, and confidence. You become centered, strong, and stable in yourself.

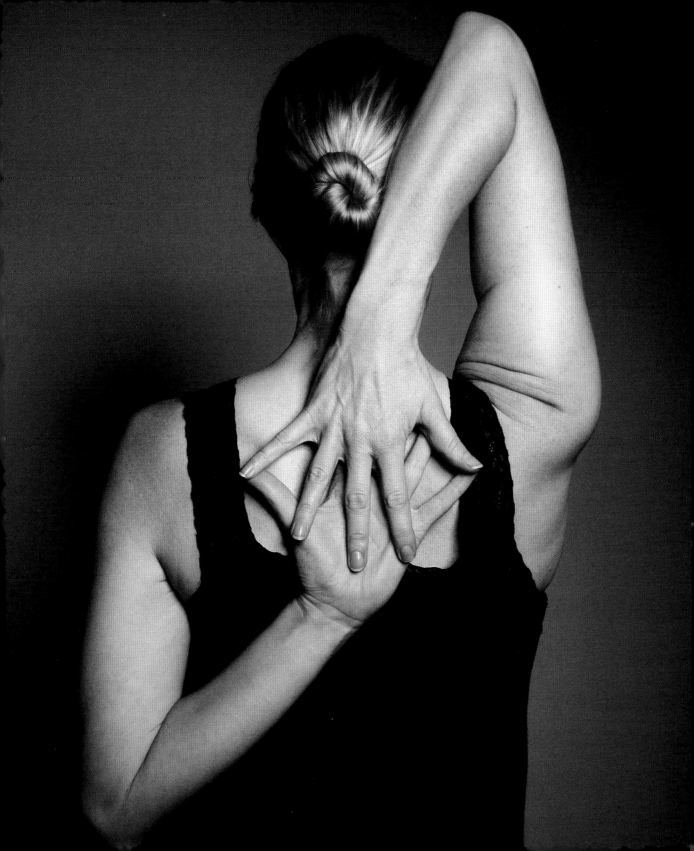

CHAPTER 5

Yoga Poses

What is absolutely of most importance in the practicing of asanas is the posture, the gaze (*drishti*) and the breathing. In the programs that follow, I have designed sequences of different types of yoga poses that can be divided into standing poses, forward bends, back bends, arm balances, seated twists, and restorative poses. The different positions are divided into "families" that train and stimulate different parts of the body. For a complete practice, you need a balanced composition of all of them. Here, I first explain the different types of positions before they are presented in more detail, so that you know the function of the different poses. In the final section of the book, I have put together a number of sequences that give you the exact practice you wish for or need the most at a specific moment.

Standing Poses

Standing poses develop strength and power. They help us to create better physical posture, help us mentally to greater self-confidence, and help us with balance, presence, and commitment. Standing poses require our full attention on the balance between relaxing and tensing our muscles.

EFFECTS:

- Stabilizes joints, strengthens and balances the muscles in the feet, ankles, knees, and hips
- Develops support and strength in the pelvis, enhances endurance, and stimulates circulation in the torso
- Strengthen the pelvic floor muscles and exercise the muscles in the pelvis
- Balance our mind and ground us
- In good posture they reduce pressure on the heart, balance the muscles of the chest and upper back, and strengthen the shoulder and neck muscles
- Increase focus and the ability of attention, especially the balancing postures

Forward Bends

Forward bends calm the nervous system and mind, and are more introspective in comparison to the more extroverted and dynamic backward bends.

Forward bends soften muscular tension around the spinal column and the back of the legs, which allows increased vitality in the entire backside of the body.

In forward bends, we want to lengthen the spine to create space between each vertebra in the spine, which stimulates the nerves around the spine, reduces compression, and nourishes the large dorsal nerve.

Forward bends in conjunction with attentive and active yoga breathing stimulates the liver, kidneys, pancreas, and intestines. The back muscles become stronger and the agility of leg muscles and tendons increases. Be careful not to force your back into something it is not ready for! Keep in mind that when you bend forward, you fold at the hip (groin), and not at the waist. This provides better agility and

NAMES OF POSES

In yoga, the traditional Sanskrit names of the poses are used as often as the English names. However, some poses, which are modern variations of traditional poses, do not have Sanskrit names. Then it may happen that the pose has an English name, simply because this is the most acknowledged in yoga today.

Yin yoga seeks for other qualities than what more active and flowing types of yoga seek. Therefore they have different names for the same poses. These poses also have other names and no traditional names in Sanskrit.

creates room for the abdominal muscles to work in order to keep the spine in a correct position. Be aware if you lose your breath or if it feels strained, then you have pushed too hard and gone too far, or failed to move into the pose with a good posture. Start from the beginning and try not to allow your ambitions and pretensions to push you too far.

EFFECTS:
- Strengthens the bones
- The spinal muscles are stretched and extended
- Increased circulation in the back and in the chest
- Balances our mind and grounds energy
- Reduces emotional stress

Back Bends

Backward bends are asanas that open up and turn the body and mind toward the world. They expand the thorax and help to release tensions in the front and the upper thoracic spine as well as strengthen the muscles in the area between the ribs, in the shoulders, and belly. Make sure that the backward bend is concentrated in the thoracic spine and not in the lumbar spine, by creating length in all postures.

EFFECTS:
- Increases mobility in the thoracic spine
- Strengthens the spinal muscles
- Increases circulation in the stomach and lungs
- Revitalizes tired legs
- Revitalizes and increases the energy in the body and mind
- Reduces fatigue and stress

Arm Balances

All balancing poses stimulate the cerebellum, the part of the brain that controls how the body works in motion, maintains physical balance, and keeps unconscious movements equilibrated. Once you achieve better balance in a posture it becomes easier to rely on other forces, such as gravity, in order to advance in the practice and consequently move deeper into the yoga positions. The body learns to conserve its own energy and becomes more flexible and you get a greater mobility and strength in movements. The arm balances also develop a balanced mind through which to face life.

EFFECTS:
- Strengthens the arms, shoulders, and wrists
- Increases circulation in the upper body
- Balances the nervous system
- Reduces stress and emotional anxiety
- Enhances patience and endurance
- Relieves depression

Rotating Poses

Rotations, or twists, are effective ways to strengthen the spine. Each yoga program should contain at least one rotation, favorably after the seated forward and back bends. Rotations should always be performed with caution and good alignment of the spine so you don't go beyond what your body actually allows. These asanas strengthen and balance the abdominal and back muscles and also stimulate the spinal nerves positively. Most of the rotations activate the area around the navel. This means that the pancreas, kidneys, stomach, small intestine, liver, and gallbladder are stimulated and that there is increased circulation in the muscle tissue in this area. Therefore, these asanas have a great overall effect on your health and vitality.

EFFECTS:

- Grounding, helps to eliminate toxins as well as stabilize the hips and pelvis
- Strengthens the spine muscles, the abdominal and chest muscles, shoulders, and neck
- Increases the ability to concentrate
- Sharpens the mind and the intellect

Restorative Poses

The resting poses create maximum relaxation for the body and mind. Sometimes tools such as blankets, blocks, and solid pillows or bolsters are used to remove all unnecessary pressure on the joints as much as possible. The resting positions should be at the end of any yoga program and are especially beneficial as a sole practice for those who are stressed, emotional, feeling weak, or pregnant.

EFFECTS:

- Creates space for increased stress relief and relaxation
- Boosts the oxygenation of the body and the blood supply to the brain
- Lowers blood pressure
- Calms the nervous system
- Lowers the level of stress in the body and mind
- Increases circulation and metabolism

YIN YOGA

Yin yoga uses the same basic poses as regular yoga but here, you work with a different approach in the practice. The purpose is neither to flex nor stretch your muscles, but rather to put a natural pressure on the muscle and bone to achieve greater elasticity in the connective tissue, balance mobility in the joints, and allow greater oxygen flow to the muscles when the tension eases.

Yin yoga practice counteracts mental and physical stress and is a great way to strengthen the mind, increase breathing capacity, and build meditation practice.

When you do yin yoga, strive for a good posture in the lumbar spine while in a seated position so that you do not slouch too much.

Use your breathing to practice relaxing your legs, shoulders, and face, and feel heavy against the mat.

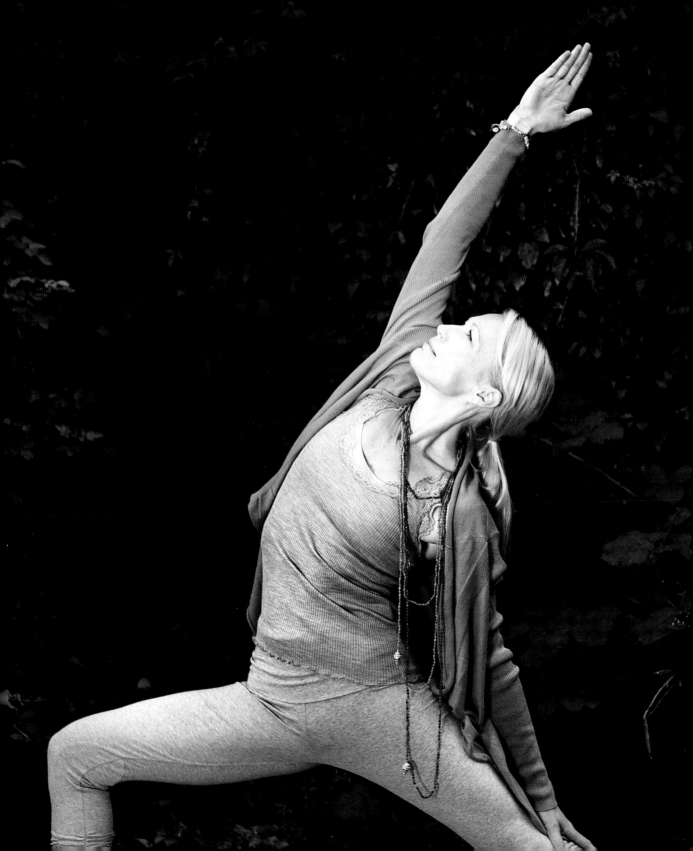

Standing Poses

Tadasana

The Mountain Pose is the blueprint not only for all standing poses but for all yoga poses because here, basic alignment is developed and practiced.

GETTING INTO THE POSE

Stand with your feet hip width apart, point your toes straight forward. Lift all ten toes, put them back down one by one, and press the floor away from you with your feet. Feel how the front of the thighs activates. Move the sitz bones toward your heels and suck your lower belly in, pushing it against the spine. Lift the sternum up toward your chin, widen the collar bones, and feel how your spine stretches. Soften your shoulders and let the back crown of your head lift upward. Steady, soft breaths in *ujjayi*.

GAZE: Follow the bridge of your nose forward to a fixed point on the floor.

TIP: Place a block in between your thighs if you can't balance well, have a knee injury, or suffer from low blood pressure.

BENEFITS:
- Improves balance
- Creates balance in the spine, hips and legs, and in the whole body if the movement is performed correctly
- Increases stability and strengthens the thighs, knees, and ankles
- Helps to focus the mind

Arms Up Pose

Urdhva hastasana

A really great chest opener that also facilitates breathing. Strive to concentrate your breathing toward the back of the body.

GETTING INTO THE POSE:

Stand in Mountain Pose. Inhale and lift your arms outwards and upward. Aim your thumbs backwards, lower your shoulders, soften the shoulder blades, and lift the sternum. Exhale out and lower your arms again.

GAZE: Straight ahead.

Chair Pose

Utkatasana

In *Utkatasana* we strengthen the muscles of the back, arms, legs, and heart and the diaphragm is stimulated.

GETTING INTO THE POSE:

From Mountain Pose, slowly bend your knees and distribute your weight evenly on your feet. Draw your sitz bones back and down and soften your tailbone downward. Sense the lower abdominal muscles activating for stability in the lumbar spine. Lift your arms forward and gently up and stretch your fingers gently. Hold your arms shoulder width apart, or let your palms meet.

GAZE: Up toward your hands or in front of you on the floor.

BENEFITS:

- Stretches and stabilizes the ankles, calves, thighs, and spine
- Improves posture and balance in the legs
- Strengthens the back and the abdominal muscles
- Develops flexibility in the chest
- Prevents stiffness in the shoulders and chest
- Stimulates the abdominal internal organs, the diaphragm, and heart due to the stretching of the spine and the force of the legs
- Creates internal heat, *agni*, which means digestive fire in Sanskrit.

Rotated Chair Pose

Parivrtta utkatasana

This pose is grounding, calming, and strengthens the legs and spine. Starting from the Chair Pose, put your hands together in front of your chest. Inhale and gently rotate your upper body to the right. Place your left elbow on the outer side of your right leg. Lengthen your spine and fix your gaze on a rearward point. Hold the pose for at least four breaths and then switch sides. Finish with the Standing Forward Bend.

GAZE: On a rearward point on the ground, floor, or mat.

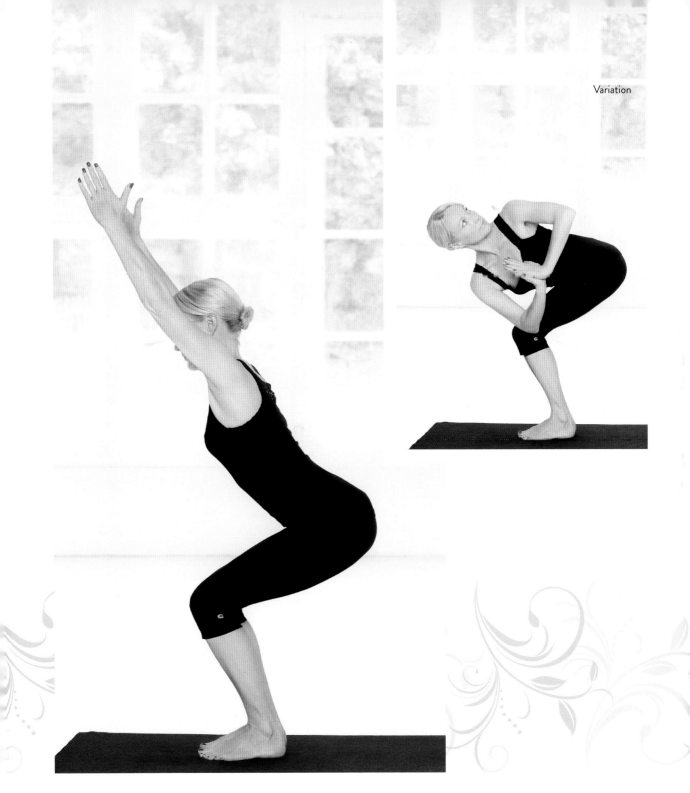

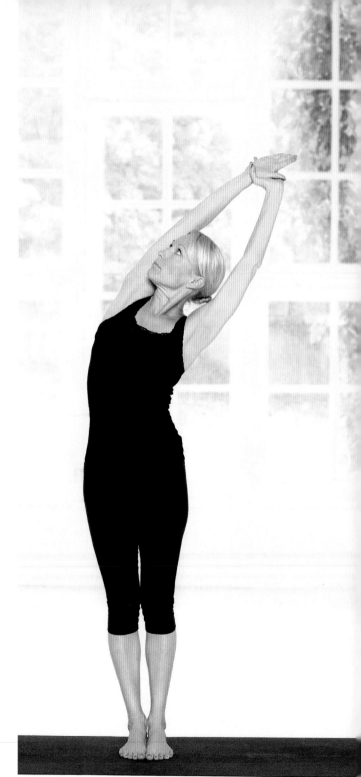

Swaying Palm Tree Pose

Tiriyaka tadasana

The Swaying Palm Tree Pose is an energizing exercise that is beneficial for the breath. It stretches the sides of the chest, the shoulders, and the muscles between the ribs while building stability in the midsection.

GETTING INTO THE POSE:

Starting from the Mountain Pose, stretch up one arm and continue stretching until you feel that you are stretching the side of your chest. Activate your legs by pressing your feet into the mat. If there is room, let your hand grip the opposite wrist and gently stretch upward. Focus on an upward direction rather than bending to the side.

GAZE: Up, or down if you have neck problems.

Standing Forward Bend

Uttanasana

A grounding and calming pose.

GETTING INTO THE POSE:

From the Mountain Pose: Inhale and lift your sternum
and gently draw your sitz bones to your heels. Exhale
and tilt your pelvis forward so that it is pointing toward
your feet. Slightly bend the knees and push the floor away
from you with your feet until you feel that the front of
your legs activate. Relax your back more and more as well
as your neck and shoulders to the best of your ability.

GAZE: Toward the floor.

GETTING OUT OF THE POSE:

On exhalation, bend your legs and on inhalation roll up
vertebra by vertebra.

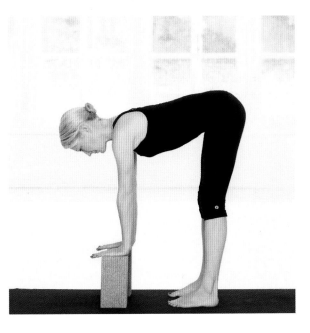

Shoulder Stretch

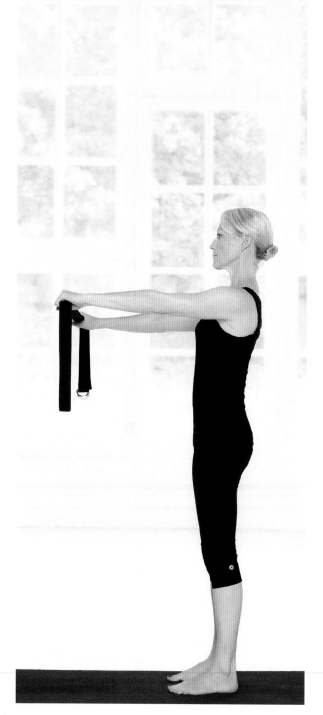

Stand in the Mountain Pose and hold a strap or a rope
stretched between your hands. Straighten your arms and
lift your chest.

Inhale and raise your arms in front of you until they
are above your head. On exhalation, proceed slowly
backward and downward. If you bend your arms and lift
your shoulders, keep your hands wider apart to create
more space in your shoulder. Then, on inhalation, go
back and lift your arms upward behind you, above your
head, and in front of you on exhalation. If you arch your
back, place a block between your thighs and squeeze
your thighs gently against the block to activate the inner
thigh muscles, the pelvic floor, and the abdominal muscles to support your lower back.

GAZE: In front of you on the floor.

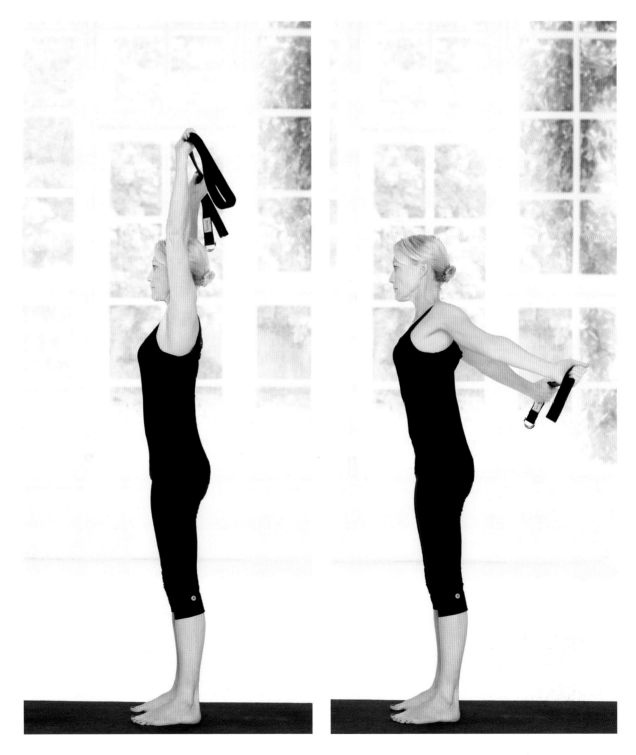

The Cat/Cow

Marjariasana/Bitiliasana

GETTING INTO THE POSE:
Kneel on all fours with your shoulders straight above
your wrists and your hips above your knees. Inhale, draw
your chest forward, slide your shoulder blades back, and
arch your back, with your eyes focused forward. Exhale
and gently round your back like a cat. Focus on finding
a stretch between your shoulder blades. Inhale and lift
your chest and gaze upward, exhale and aim your gaze
toward your body.

GAZE: Forward, then toward your body.

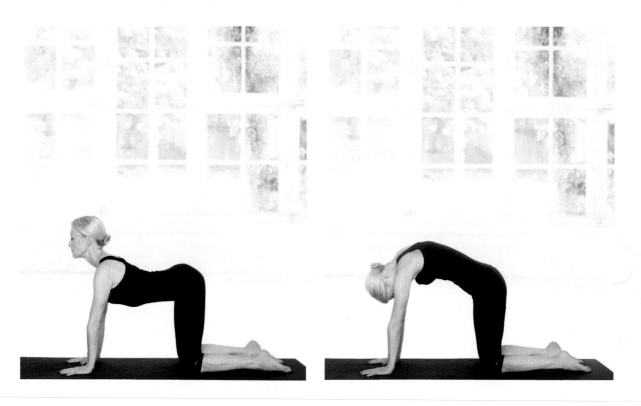

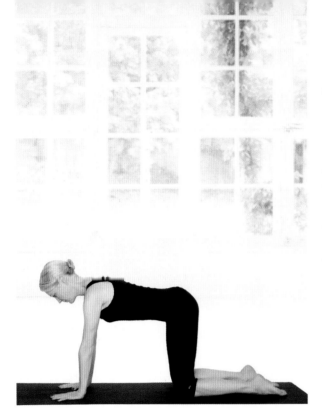

Tiger Pose

Vyaghrasana

Strengthens the spine, stabilizes the hip, and increases circulation in the torso, shoulders, and neck.

GETTING INTO THE POSE:

Kneel on all fours and breathe in an even pace. Spread your fingers and press your palms against the floor. Your wrist, shoulders, hips, and knees should be in a straight line. Stretch out your left arm in front of you and your right leg straight back behind you.

Activate your right arm and left leg muscles by pushing your palms and shins downward, into the mat. Make sure that the hip bones point downward toward the floor. Repeat the same thing on the opposite side.

GAZE: Between your hands.

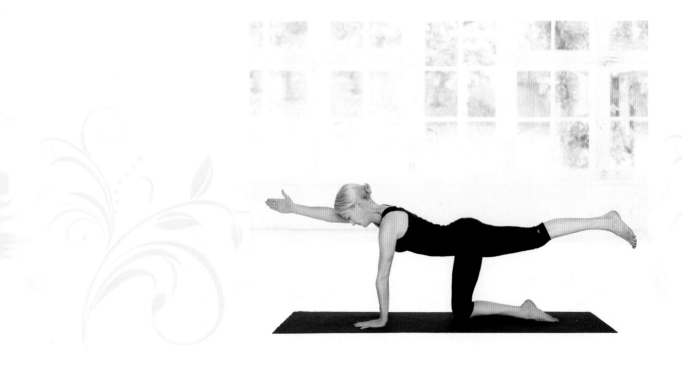

Reverse Warrior Pose

Surya virabhadrasana

A variation of the Warrior Pose that opens up
the side of the body. From Warrior 2, if your
right leg is aimed forward and bent, lift up
your right arm and lower your left hand and
rest it lightly on the left thigh.

GAZE: Up on your hand.

Dragon Pose

A classic yin yoga pose which is a variant of the Warrior Pose or Lizard Pose in yang yoga.

GETTING INTO THE POSE:

From all fours or the Downward Dog, take a step forward with your left foot and let your upper body rest on your thigh. Feel a slight stretch in the right thigh and the front of the hip. Hold the pose, breathe, and try to be "heavy" and relaxed.

GAZE: Eyes closed.

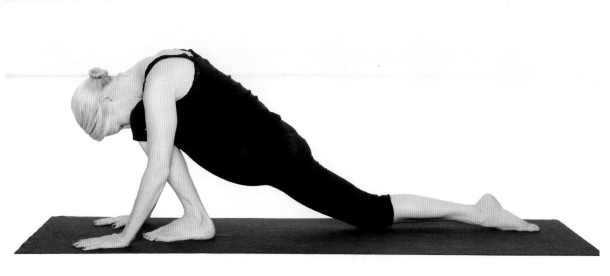

"STRETCH THE SPINE BY LEADING
YOUR STERNUM UP
AND SOFTEN YOUR SHOULDERS."

Crescent Moon Pose

Anjaneyasana

Low lunge, hip stretchers (modification). The Crescent Moon Pose is often called just the Crescent Pose.

GETTING INTO THE POSE:

1. From the Downward Dog: On exhalation, step forward with your right leg between your hands. Bend your leg and place your knee above your heel. Stretch your rear leg and press your toes into the mat. Press down your front foot into the mat in order to create stability in the pose. Stretch the spine by leading your sternum up and softening your shoulders.

Now activate your leg muscles, lift up your upper body, and stretch your arms upward. Find support in the abdominal muscles by gently drawing your sitz bones down and hip bones up. Breathe deep. Change sides and repeat the movement.

2. Simplified Crescent Moon Pose. From Uttanasana: Place your fingertips on the floor or your hands on two blocks, step backwards with your right leg, and in a low lunge get up on your fingertips.

Stretch your rear leg and press your toes into the mat. Press your front foot into the mat to create stability in the pose. Stretch the spine by leading your sternum forward and soften down your shoulders.

Now activate your leg muscles and stretch your arms upward. Find support in the abdominal muscles by gently pulling your navel in toward the spine.

Change sides and repeat the movement.

GAZE: Down and forward or up if you stand in the Crescent Moon Pose.

46

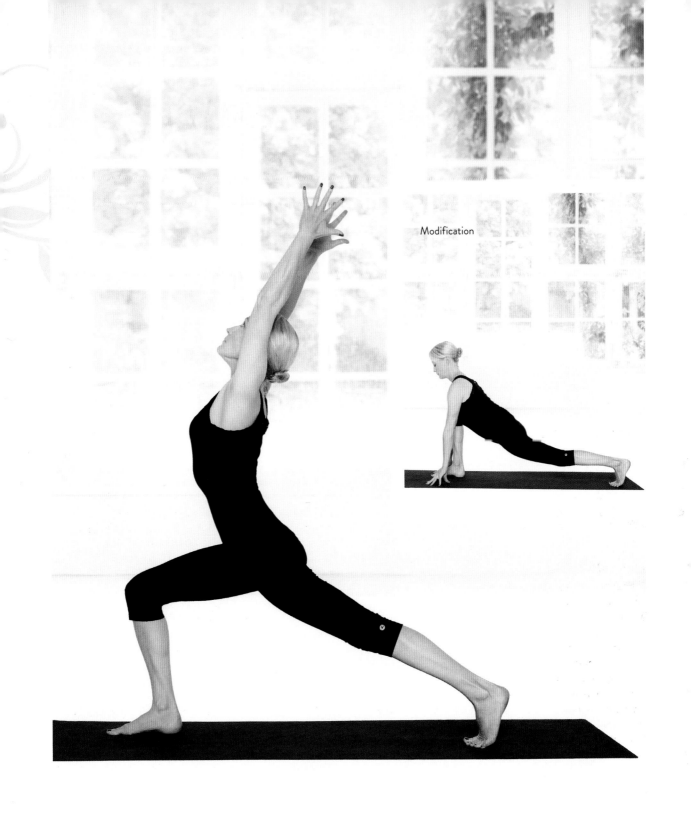

Modification

Warrior Pose 1, 2, 3

Virabhadrasana 1, 2, 3

The Warrior Poses are powerful poses that disengage a large amount of prana in the body, especially from the hips, legs, and chest. According to yoga philosophy they increase our inner fire, *agni*, and stimulates digestion.

GETTING INTO THE POSE:

1. WARRIOR POSE 1

From the Downward Dog: On inhalation, step forward with your right foot between your hands. Lower the rear sole of the foot behind you onto the mat in a 45-degree angle and try to make sure all ten toes come into contact with the mat. Stretch your back leg and press your foot down into the mat.

Lift your upper body by pushing off with the front foot (press your heel into the mat so that the front and back thighs are activated, this provides better stability in the pelvis) and strive to lift your chest upward. Hands shoulder width apart or palms together above your head, depending on the flexibility in your shoulder area. From Uttanasana or the Mountain Pose: Inhale and step backward with one foot. Then proceed as above. Change sides and repeat the movement.

GAZE: Forward or upward if your neck is sore.

2. WARRIOR POSE 2

From the Mountain Pose: Inhale and on exhalation, take a big step backward with your right leg. Turn your rear foot 90 degrees and stretch your leg. Make sure that the front lower leg keeps a straight line from your knee to your heel and that you activate your legs by pushing your toes and your heels down into the mat. Lift up your arms and stretch them out to the sides of each leg parallel to the floor. Change sides and repeat the movement.

GAZE: On your hand in front of you.

3. WARRIOR POSE 3

From Warrior 1 or Crescent Moon Pose: Move the weight to the front foot. Extend your chest and let the hip be parallel with the floor. Place your hands on two blocks in front of you or sweep your arms forward or outward. Stretch the leg you are standing on as well as the stretched leg as you aim your chest forward. Steady breaths.

Change sides and repeat the movement.

GAZE: Down on the floor in front of you.

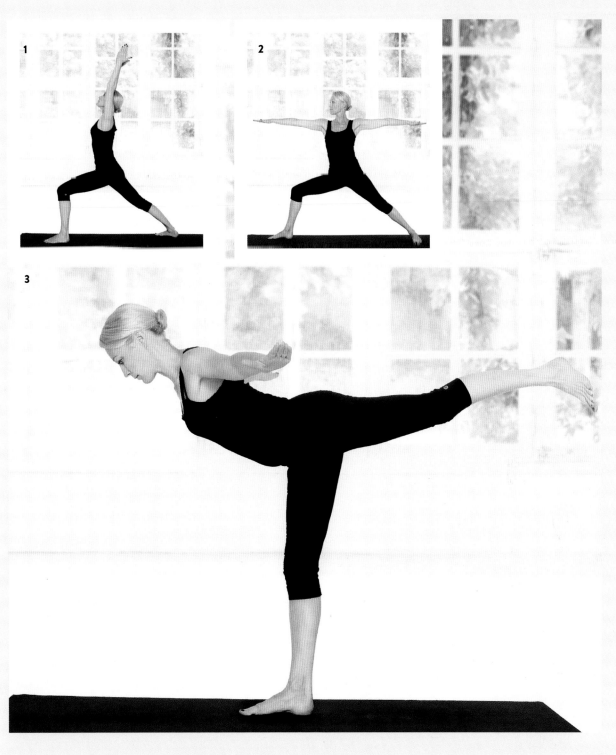

Downward-Facing Dog Pose

Adho Mukha Svanasana

This is a full body stretch. Circulation is increased, muscles are strengthened and shaped in legs, arms, stomach, and shoulders, fatigue is counteracted, and vitality is increased in the body's organs and muscles. The Downward Dog is one of the poses in the traditional sun salutation sequence. It is however a great asana by itself. A good way to strengthen the whole body is to stand in the pose for 1–3 minutes. Then bend your knees and rest in the Child's Pose.

GETTING INTO THE POSE:

Kneel on all fours with your hands right beneath your shoulders and your knees beneath the hip. Spread your fingers and press your entire palm down into the mat. Curl your toes into the mat. Exhale and lift up your knees, draw the sitz bones back, and slowly push your buttocks upward. Push the mat away from you with your hands and extend your arms while your back is stretched. Keep your head between your arms and gently pull your navel toward the spine.

During the same exhalation, try also to stretch your legs a little bit by activating the front of your thigh muscles and push off with the big toes without lifting your heels. Slightly extend your knees. The heels strive toward the floor. Stretch your arms and push your palms down. Spread out your shoulder blades. Breathe.

GAZE: For beginners, between the legs. For more advanced, squinting toward the navel (without moving your head).

NOTE: The most important thing is not for the heels to come down to the floor, but to extend the back and relieve the shoulders. If this means that you have to push off the floor with your hands and bend your knees, I would recommend it!

"FATIGUE IS COUNTERACTED AND VITALITY IS INCREASED IN THE BODY'S ORGANS AND MUSCLES."

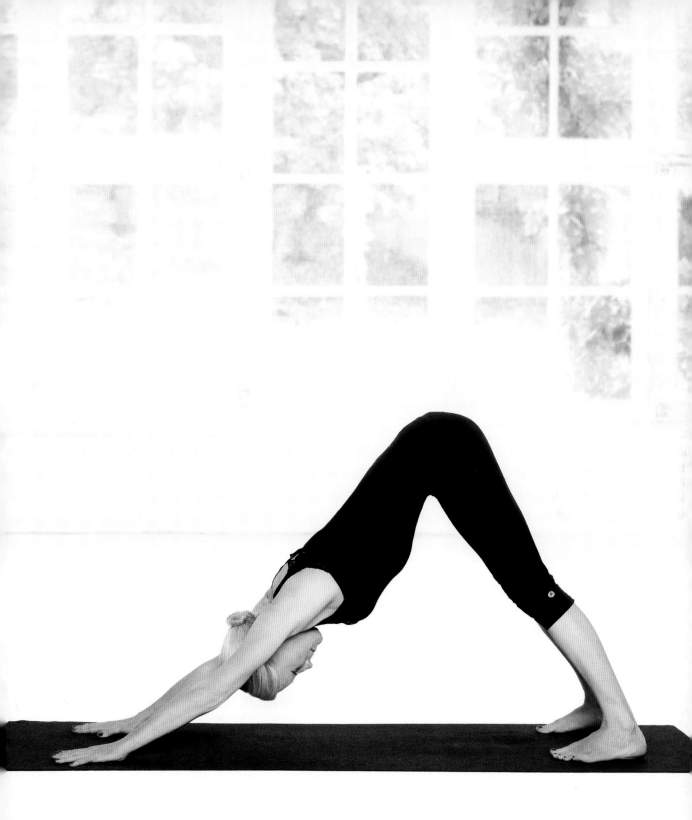

Wide-Legged Forward Bend

Prasarita padottanasana

The Wide-Legged Forward Bend strengthens the leg muscles, increases flexibility in the spine, increases lung capacity, and helps you breathe more deeply.

GETTING INTO THE POSE:

From the Mountain Pose: Step wide apart, extend your arms, and stretch your legs. Watch the position of your feet; your toes should point straight forward and your heels straight back. This is to protect your knees and hips. Stretch your legs. Inhale and stretch, lengthening your spine. Gaze forward, exhale, and let your eyes follow your nose forward and downward and fold your back down toward the floor, stopping halfway.

1. If you feel tightness in your legs or back, you can benefit from placing your hands on two blocks (modified version). Lengthen your back on each inhalation, exhale, and stay in the position. Let the weight rest in the front part of the foot.

GAZE: Down toward the floor.

2. Place your hands on the floor between your legs, fingers pointing straight down. Inhale and stretch the spine, exhale, and fold forward deeper. Stop and breathe. Draw your sitz bones back and lengthen your back on inhaling, exhale and fold your body over toward your legs. Relax your shoulders, arms, and face. Keep equal weight on your legs and if you come down with your head to the floor avoid bending your neck, strive to keep a straight line in the cervical spine. Place your tongue lightly on the palate to activate the anterior neck muscles which stabilize your neck.

GAZE: Down toward the floor.

3. If you want to give yourself a challenge you can interlace your fingers behind your back and lift your hands up toward the ceiling while stretching your back. Then, separate your hands and lower them to the mat again.

GAZE: Between your feet.

GETTING OUT OF THE POSE:

Inhale and extend your back forward, exhale and come back again. Bend your knees and put your legs together. Keep your legs bent and *drishti* onto the floor. Inhale, feel the support in your legs and stomach and roll up vertebra by vertebra (relax your shoulders and neck) until you are standing with your back straight in the Mountain Pose.

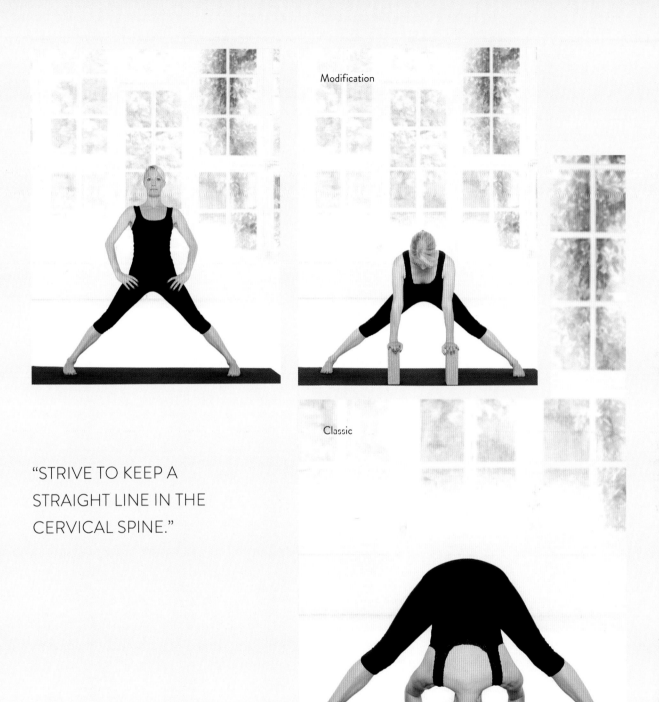

Modification

Classic

"STRIVE TO KEEP A
STRAIGHT LINE IN THE
CERVICAL SPINE."

Child's Pose

Balasana

Increases resilience of body and mind, calms the brain, and reduces stress and fatigue.

GETTING INTO THE POSE:

Kneel on all fours, with your knees hip width apart. Lower your buttocks toward your heels and lengthen your back as much as possible. Rest your forehead against the floor. Let your neck be long and relaxed. Also relax your jaw, shoulders, and neck. Let your arms rest in front of you (or if you want to stretch your shoulders and chest, put your arms on your side with your palms facing upward). Relax your entire body and feel your breath in the thoracic spine. Broaden your chest while inhaling and soften it on exhalation.

GAZE: Eyes closed.

"RELAX IN YOUR ENTIRE BODY AND FEEL YOUR BREATH IN THE THORACIC SPINE."

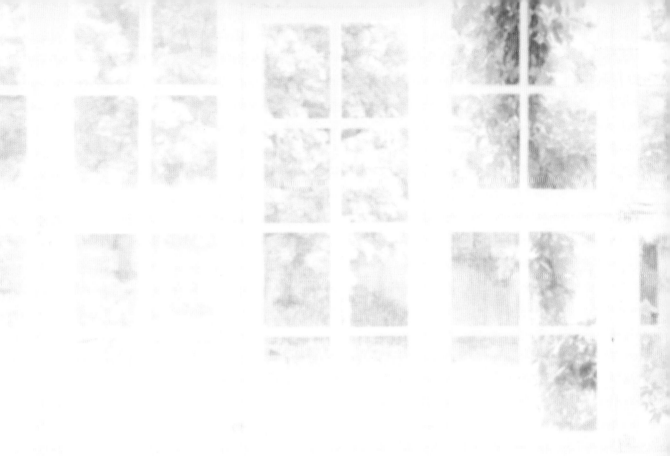

Head-to-Knee Pose

Janu sirsasana

Stretches the back muscles, shoulders, back of the thighs, and groin.
Improves digestion and can alleviate menopausal symptoms.

GETTING INTO THE POSE:

Sit up straight with your legs stretched out straight in front of you. Inhale and
lengthen your back and aim your chest upward. Slowly lead your left foot
toward the right inside of your calf or thigh. Hold a rope or a strap with both
hands around your front foot or hold it with your hands around your calf or
foot. Try to stretch and lengthen your back (to avoid compression in the lumbar), allowing you to get more activity in the front of your legs while inhaling.

GAZE: On your toes.

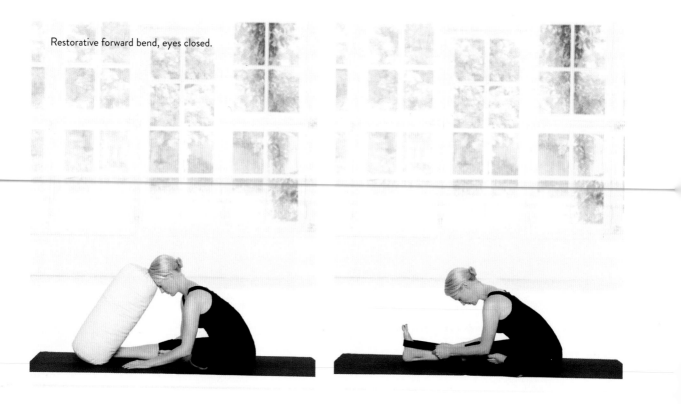

Restorative forward bend, eyes closed.

56

Full Forward Bend

Paschimottanasana

Helps in relaxing a stressed mind.

GETTING INTO THE POSE:

Sit up with a straight back and with your legs stretched out straight in front of you. Inhale and lengthen your back and lift your chest upward, exhale and fold forward slowly. Feel that your navel comes down before your chest does. Feel free to use a strap around your feet for better alignment in the spine or if you can reach, hold your feet or toes with your hands. Chest forward, flexed feet.

GAZE: Close your eyes or keep your gaze on your toes.

NOTE: Avoid this movement if you have trouble with your back, a herniated disc, or respiratory problems.

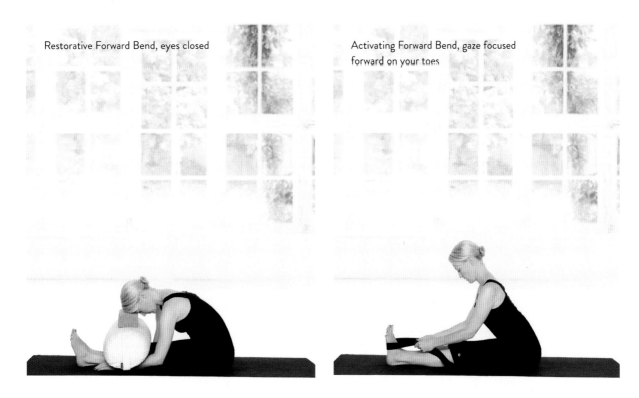

Restorative Forward Bend, eyes closed

Activating Forward Bend, gaze focused forward on your toes

Reclining Big Toe Pose

Supta Padangusthasana

A great complement if you think that the forward bends are difficult or if you have an achy lower back. This series also increases circulation in the legs and pelvis, and calms the energy of the nervous system. For a yin yoga variation of the movement you do not have to use the strap, but strive to relax in the foot a little. Hold the position for up to a few minutes in each step.

GETTING INTO THE POSE:
IN THREE STEPS:

1. Lie on your back. Stretch your right leg up toward the ceiling. Flexed feet. Hold the pose for 4–8 breaths.
2. Then, unfold your leg over to the right, keep your right side on the mat, and look at your left arm. Keep the pose for 4–8 breaths.
3. Unfold your right leg over your left leg and extend your back, look at your right hand. Keep the pose for 4–8 breaths.

GAZE: On your foot and then your arm.

1

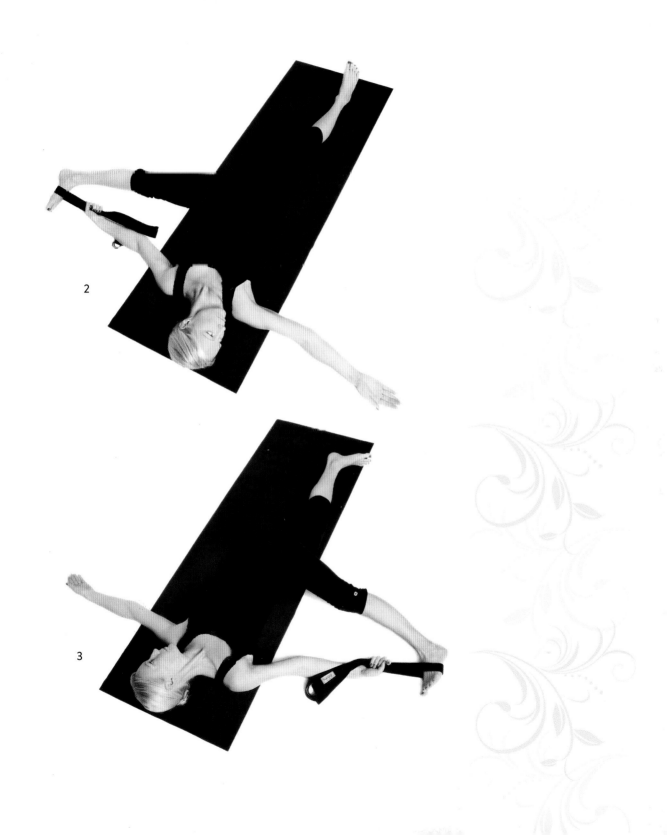

Wide-Angle Seated Forward Bend

Upavishta Konasana

Upavishta = upright, elevating

GETTING INTO THE POSE:

1. Sit with a straight back and straight legs. Keep your arms along the side of your body and next to the buttocks. Move your buttocks back a little and follow along with your hands. Breathe calmly and deeply. Straighten your back and let your legs slide apart so that they are extended in the form of a V from the hip. Draw your sitz bones to the floor and try to keep the pelvis from tilting back or forward. Allow your feet to be flexed and tighten the front thigh. Keep your toes pointing toward the ceiling. Straighten your back a little more and lift your chest.

2. Inhale and feel that you are lifting your spine off the floor by pressing the sitz bones down. Work with gravity. Focus on your breath and your posture. Keep your upper body stretched and still on inhalation and try to fold your upper body from the groin on exhalation. Make sure your back is as straight as possible all the time. Feel free to close your eyes. Stop when you feel that you have reached your limit and just breathe. Relax your shoulders.

3. When you do the restorative variation, lean your head against a bolster (see yoga practice tools on page 79). Relax your legs and feel how your body becomes heavy. Close your eyes and breathe slowly.

To get out from the pose, inhale and hold the position; on exhalation lift your back up slowly to a sitting position and gradually pull your legs back together again.

GAZE: Forward.

"IMAGINE THAT YOU HAVE A WIRE RUNNING FROM YOUR NAVEL DOWN TO THE FLOOR."

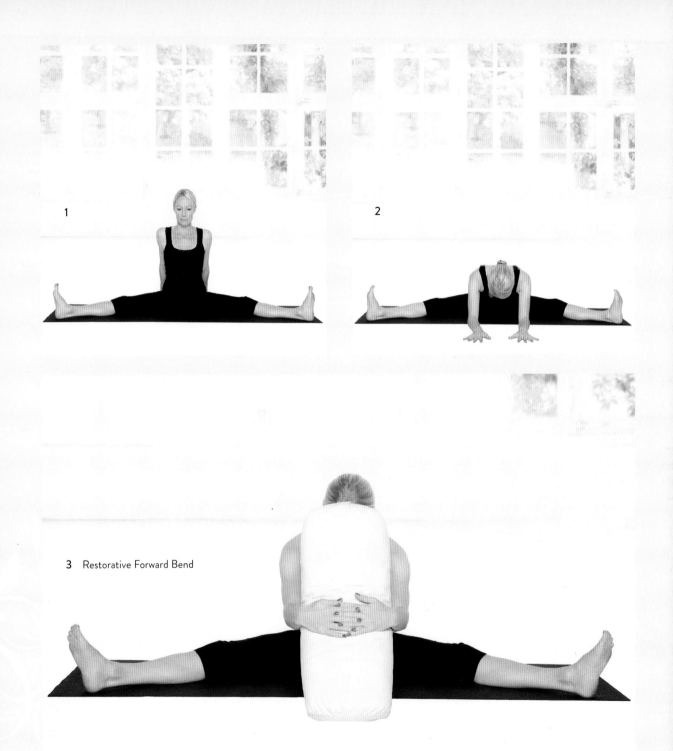

1

2

3   Restorative Forward Bend

Half Pigeon Pose

Ardha Rajakapotasana

A posture that increases circulation in the hip and lumbar, as well as the inside and the outside of the thigh. It stretches the buttock muscles and helps to release tension in the lower back. The Half Pigeon on your back is a good variant if you have knee problems. Also good for pregnant women.

GETTING INTO THE POSE:

From all fours: Inhale and place your right knee behind your right hand. Try to place your right leg at a 45 degree angle under you. If you land on your buttocks, you have gone too far for your mobility. In that case, pull your right heel against your left groin. Place your hands on each side of your leg, keeping your left leg extended straight behind you with the hip bones pointing downward. Try to maintain a steady weight above the floor. Inhale, look up and stretch your back, exhale and come down on your elbows. Keep a steady breath and try to keep your back straight and your arms relaxed. Inhale and if it feels okay, slowly walk with your hands forward. Take it easy! Stay where it says stop, close your eyes, concentrate on the area of your body where you feel stretching and pulling. Then, move to the Downward Dog Pose, stretch out and change sides.

GAZE: Eyes closed.

Half Pigeon Pose on Your Back

Supta Ardha Rajakapotasana

Lie on your back and hug your right leg toward your chest. Then, lead your left foot toward the right front thigh and place it just below your knee. Lead your left arm through the hole between your legs and grab with both hands behind your thigh. Try pressing your lower back into the mat and aim your legs toward you until you feel a stretch on the outside of your hips/buttocks. Stay like this for eight breaths before you change to the opposite leg.

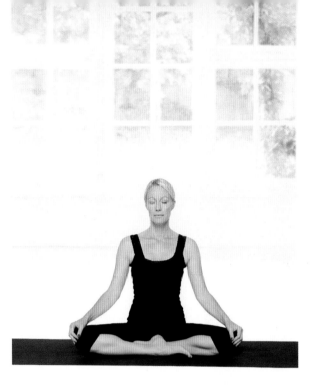

The Accomplished Pose

Siddhasana

An ideal seated position for meditation, it stabilizes the pelvis.

GETTING INTO THE POSE:

Sit on the floor, mat, or a blanket. Place your right foot with your heel in front of the pubic bone and your left heel in front of your right heel. Let your hands rest on your knees. Gently lengthen your spine. If you have sensitive knees or a sensitive lower back you can put blocks under your knees. You can also sit leaning against a wall for more stability.

GAZE: On a point on the floor in front of you.

BENEFITS:

- Calms the brain and nervous system
- Stretches the ankles and knees
- Exercises concentration

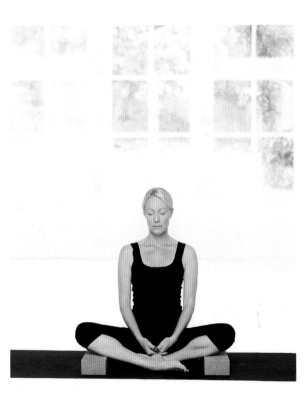

The Butterfly/ Bound Angle Pose

Baddha Konasana

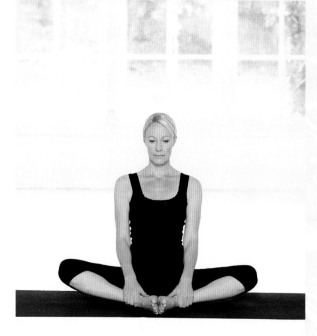

This pose will help you release tension in the lumbar and sacral spine and around the pelvis. It has a recovering and calming effect.

GETTING INTO THE POSE:

From sitting: Inhale, put the soles of your feet together and pull your heels toward your pelvis. Sit properly on both sitz bones and stretch your back. Grasp your feet, inhale, lift your sternum up, and soften in your hips and shoulders. Exhale. Work on gently folding forward with a lengthened spine and even breath.

GAZE: On the tip of your nose.

WORTH NOTING:

If you can fold your upper body over your legs without bending your back or pulling your legs up toward your ears, then lean your forehead against the floor and take eight deep breaths. Many will not be able to bring the knees down to the floor because their inner thighs are too stiff or too tense. Try to maintain a straight back and aim primarily for a good posture in your back and gradually bring your thighs down.

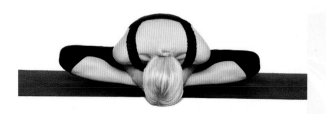

Restorative Forward Bend

Let your head drop toward the bolster and relax your shoulders. Place blocks under your knees/thighs to give the hip increased stability and to make it easier to release tension in your lower back.

Bridge Pose

Setu Bandha Sarvangasana

The variation with the block under the lower back is a more restorative option.

GETTING INTO THE POSE:

Lie on your back. Bend your knees and place your feet firmly on the floor with your heels toward your buttocks. Your feet and your knees should be hip width apart and it is important that your toes are not pointing outwards but straight forward and that your heels are pressed against your body (otherwise the knees will be overloaded). Furthermore, it is very important not to let your knees be pulled apart. Imagine that you are holding a melon that is not allowed to fall down between your knees. Try to reach your heels with your fingers or grasp your ankles.

Move your shoulder blades together and imagine that your head is gently stretched out from your shoulders.

Relax your neck and look at your navel. Inhale and rest in this position. Activate the energy in your legs and feet. Exhale and lift your buttocks off the mat and aim your hips upward as high as you can. Do not forget to press your knees against the imaginary melon. Keep in mind that the transfer is from the legs and that the navel and chest is lifted up from the shoulders (do not tighten your shoulders, here it is just the legs that are activated).

Relax your jaw and place your tongue gently against the palate. Inhale and hold the position.

GAZE: Up toward the ceiling.

GETTING OUT OF THE POSE:

Exhale as you slowly lower your hips down toward the mat. Hold with your legs all the way down. Feel how the muscles in your lower back get to relax properly.

BENEFITS:
- Increases mobility in the thoracic spine, around the shoulder blades and shoulders
- Promotes oxygenation

"FEEL HOW THE MUSCLES IN YOUR
LOWER BACK SOFTEN"

Restorative Backward Bend

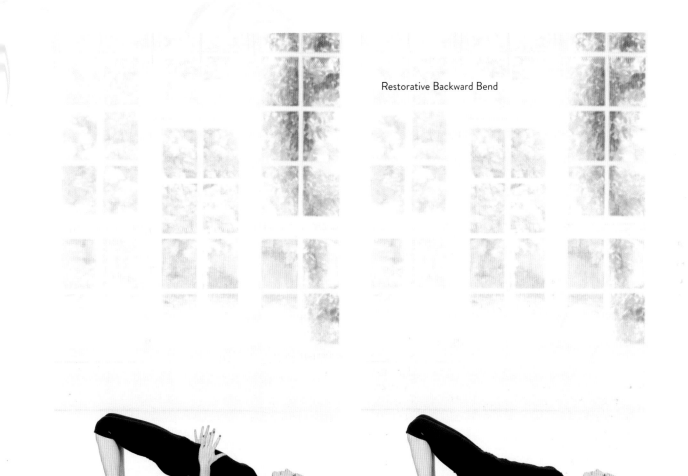

Cobra Pose

Bhujangasana

Lie on your stomach. Inhale and stretch your legs and press the feet on the mat so you can energize the legs. Press down the dorsum of your feet and let your stomach touch the mat. Focus on opening your solar plexus. Spread your fingers, bring your palms backward on the mat until you feel your shoulder blades touching. Push your palms down into the floor.

GAZE: Down, inward toward the sternum.

BENEFITS:

- Increases the mobility of the spine
- Facilitates breathing

Sphinx Pose

Lie on your stomach and relax your legs, buttocks, and lumbar spine. Place your elbows under your shoulders and your fingers forward, palms down. Move your breath to the solar plexus and stomach, and try to relax your legs and buttocks. Hold this position for four to eight breaths to increase circulation, or three minutes if you need to work deeper. Relax your face.

GAZE: Forward or with eyes closed.

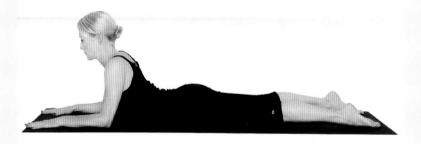

Seal Pose

From the Sphinx, extend your arms in the form of a V in front of you and stretch your arms. Let your loins, buttocks, and legs be as relaxed as possible. Breathe down in the lumbar and solar plexus.

GAZE: Forward or with eyes closed.

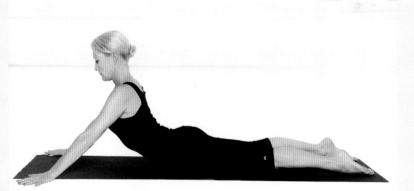

Dolphin Pose

Makarasana

The Dolphin Pose is a yoga exercise that builds up stability and strength in the upper back and activates the blood flow around the shoulders, shoulder blades, and neck. It works great as a preparation for all forearm balances and shoulder-standing asanas.

GETTING INTO THE POSE:

From the Downward Dog Pose: Stand on your forearms and place your elbows directly below your shoulders. Press your palms down, draw your collar bones apart, and soften your shoulders down the back until you feel that the chest and arm muscles increase their muscular activity. Press your forearms down and lift your hips up toward the ceiling.

GAZE: Down in front of you.

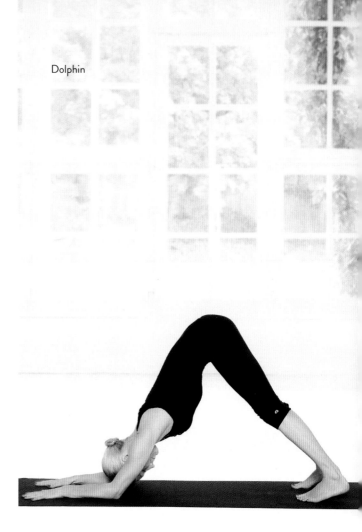

Dolphin

A VARIATION OF THE DOLPHIN:

Begin by lying down on your stomach. Stand on your forearms and place your elbows directly below your shoulders. Press your palms against a block, spread your shoulders apart, and pull your shoulder blades backwards until you feel that the arm muscles are active. Point your toes toward the mat behind you and stretch your legs. Pull your shoulder blades backwards and your chest forward and lift your hips off the mat with strong legs.

GAZE: Down on the block.

Chest and Shoulder Stretch

Anahatasana

Kneel on all fours and step forward with your arms. Lower your chest and rest your forehead on the floor (or put your forehead on a block). Keep a straight line from your hips down to your knees. Stretch your arms and let your shoulders drop down gently. Point your fingers upward, shoulder blades back, and shoulders apart; pull your navel in toward your spine and press your forearms lightly down into the floor. This is a fantastic yin yoga variation.

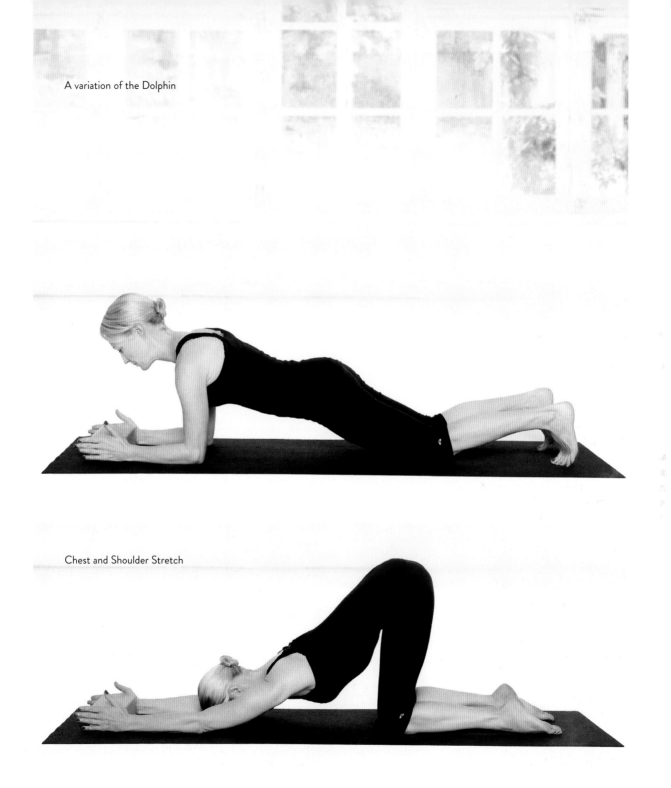

A variation of the Dolphin

Chest and Shoulder Stretch

Half Spinal Twist

Ardha Matsyendrasana

GETTING INTO THE POSE:

From sitting: Stretch your legs in front of you and straighten your back. If you need to, sit on a pillow or a folded blanket in order not to arch your back too much. Now lift your left foot over the outside of your right leg. Keep equal weight on both buttock bones. Hug your left knee with your right arm and place your left hand behind you on the floor. Let your fingers point away from your body. Inhale, straighten your back, and pull in your knee with your arm toward the right armpit. Turn your palm upward and keep the back of your hand strong. Exhale and rotate in the upper back, and look over your left shoulder. Avoid resting your body weight on the arm behind you.

Take four to eight breaths.

GETTING OUT OF THE POSE:

Inhale and come out of the pose on exhalation. Change sides and repeat.

GAZE: Aim your gaze out to the side in the rotation. If your neck feels fine, focus your gaze backward on the floor.

NOTE: If you are pregnant, you should not rotate so deep. Instead focus on lengthening the spine.

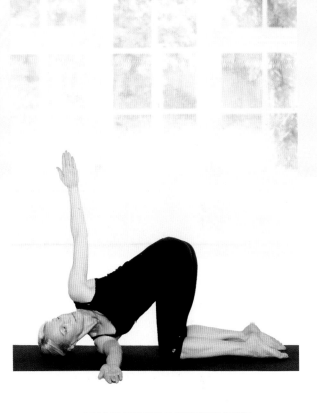

A VARIANT FOR THE SEATED ROTATION POSE:

Sewing Thread Rotation

Kneel on all fours and bring the weight of your lower body over to your left leg. Bring your right arm through the space between your arm and leg. Put your right arm down on the floor, palm up. Let your shoulder blades be pulled back so that the neck stretches gently. Then, lift your left arm toward the ceiling or rest your left arm on your lower back. Strive to steer your breath more to the thoracic posterior parts. Stay like this for 4–8 breaths and come back slowly to all fours before repeating on the opposite side.

Reclining Spine Twist

Shava Udarakarshanasana

An exercise that reduces tension in the lower back and allows the spine to get back to the neutral original position after Backward Bends. This pose has a calming effect on the nervous system and prepares the body well for relaxation.

Lie down on your back, bend your legs, and fold them to the right, stretch out your arms and turn your face toward your left arm so that there is a twist in the spine. Then change sides.

NOTE: If you experience uncomfortable sensations in your lower back, place a blanket or a pillow between your thighs.

GAZE: Toward your arm.

Legs Up Against the Wall

Viparita Karani

This movement increases blood flow in the pelvis, chest, neck, and face. This exercise has a restorative effect on the nervous system and increases the blood supply to the brain. A perfect asana for relaxation. Lie on your back with a bolster (or a regular pillow or blanket) under your lower back with your legs bent or stretched up against a wall. Ensure that the bolster is located under your lower back. Breathe long, deep breaths and stay preferably in this position until you feel an increased mental and physical calm.

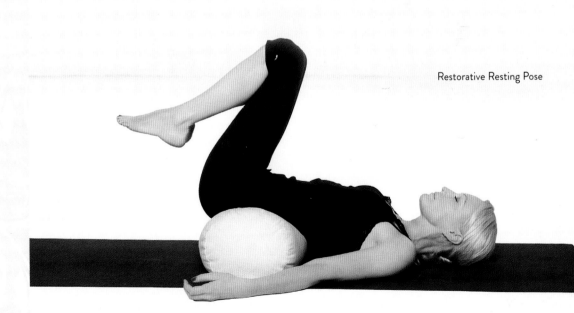

Restorative Resting Pose

Corpse Pose

Savasana

Sava = corpse/dead

When you relax in the Corpse Pose your mind and body rests. Feel free to put a blanket over your stomach. If you put a bolster under your knees, the tension in the lower back reduces.

GETTING INTO THE POSE:

Lie fully extended with your arms along your body. Lower your lower back into the floor, shoulder blades together, pull your arms down toward your feet, and lift up your chin a little. Keep your legs hip width apart and let your feet fall out in different directions, and turn your palms up toward the ceiling. Take a deep breath and close your eyes. Relax. Let your breaths be long and deep.

Feel your body sinking into the mat and let go of all thoughts and feelings. Keep breathing calmly while you try to relax every muscle, including your face, hands, and feet. Try to focus on the diaphragm. Each time you exhale, release more and more stress and tension in your muscles. Now focus on your feet, tighten them as you inhale and relax them as you exhale. Do the same thing with your hands and feel how you relax more and more in the rest of your body. Now try to relax your face and breathe deeply.

Reward yourself with a few minutes of nice rest and lie like this for a couple of minutes, preferably 7–15 minutes.

GAZE: Eyes closed.

"FEEL YOUR BODY SINKING INTO THE MAT AND SLOWLY LET GO OF ALL THOUGHTS AND FEELINGS."

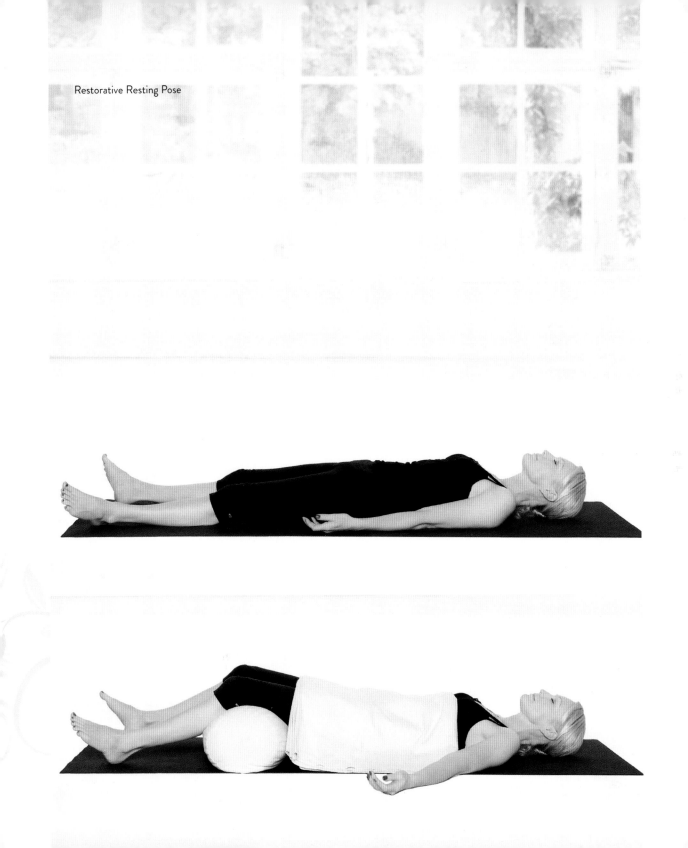

Restorative Resting Pose

CHAPTER 6

Yoga Flows

Each of the classes presented here, which you can practice at home, are of different character so that you can choose according to your needs. Maybe you want to have a quieter and softer session, or you want a practice that is more dynamic. Adapt your practice to the needs you have at the moment. Sessions 1, 3, 5, and 6 are more active and abundant (yang yoga) for days when you need to feel more stability in your body, get the circulation going, and raise the energy level in body and mind.

Sessions 2, 4, and 7 have more of the yin yoga character, where you stimulate the connective tissue in your body. These sessions have a relaxing, restoring, and up-building effect on the body. For those of you who are used to practicing yoga, I suggest that you use the session lay-ups as an inspiration for your own practice, and you should feel free to adapt them to your own needs and circumstances.

Have you just started practicing yoga? I advise you to take it step by step. Perform each of the programs a couple of times and focus on synchronizing your breathing with the exercise. In the beginning it will feel challenging. As a general rule it is said that it takes twelve weeks of regular exercise for 15 minutes a day before one gets into a routine. The practice should not hurt or be painful. In this case, step back or stop the pose. However, there can be a kind of "feel-good pain" pulling in the muscles, and this is perfectly okay and not dangerous.

> **NOTE:**
>
> If you're unsure of whether you should perform some of the exercises, consult your doctor, a physical therapist, or an experienced yoga teacher.
>
> If you are pregnant, you should be cautious and avoid twists, laying on your stomach, and dynamic jumps between poses, and I also recommend you not to go further or deeper into the poses than you could before you became pregnant.

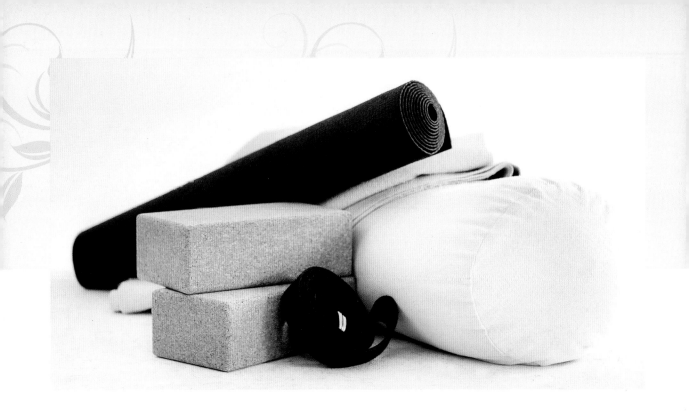

USEFUL TOOLS FOR YOGA PRACTICE:

In order to facilitate and/or deepen and create a greater impact in practice, there are different tools.

YOGA MAT – to get a better grip in postures. A rug or other type of mat works well, but it is not as stable.

BLANKET – to sit on, cover yourself with, or use as a support under the knees in kneeling positions or under the bottom in sitting positions.

BOLSTER – long, round pillow that helps recompress pressure of the joints, to lie on and to be used as support in many poses. A pillow or something similar is also okay.

BLOCK – can create a better posture. It's also good to use when you need more movement space for joints and spine, or a relief. If you do not have a yoga block, use a thick book with a ribbon or something similar around it.

YOGA STRAP – provides better stability for the joints and helps you get a better reach in certain positions. A bathrobe sash or another type of strap works great as well.

EYE BAGS – for increased stress relief and relaxation effect. If you do not have an eye bag, you can put a soft shirt or another cloth over your eyes.

MUSIC – If playing good music helps you become more peaceful and allows you to relax, it's an excellent tool.

TIP!

In order to know how long you should lie in relaxation or stay in a position that you are encouraged to stay in for a couple of minutes, I recommend using an egg timer. You can use your smartphone or download a timer app with a pleasant sound.

Spine and Hips

This is a get-started practice for beginners, or for those who want a more general basic session. Start by lying on your back and try to focus on taking long, deep breaths to let your body calm down. Thus even your mind will be calmed and you will be less stressed on starting the movements.

Now follows a laying series to increase circulation in the legs and hips. Then, get into the Bridge Pose and keep it for 8 breaths. Slowly lower your back, lift your legs inwards toward your chest, and hug your legs. Rock from side to side and then up to a sitting position and proceed to stand on all fours. Hold the following positions for 4 breaths each (longer if you want a session longer than 15 minutes). Afterwards, when you get down on your back in the Corpse Pose, try to lie down for three minutes.

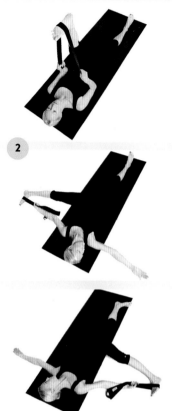

1. Corpse Pose, 8 breaths.
2. Lying Leg Flexor, 4 breaths in each step, both sides.
3. Bridge Pose. Hug your knees and then roll up to all fours.
4. Tiger Pose.
5. Cat/Cow Pose.
6. Downward-Facing Dog Pose.
7. Lying face down, Cobra Pose.
8. Child's Pose.
9. Downward-Facing Dog Pose.
10. Crescent Moon Pose, both sides.
11. Downward-Facing Dog Pose.
12. Chair Pose
13. Standing Forward Bend.
14. Corpse Pose, 3 minutes.

Lift your right leg and grab your toe or put a strap around your foot and slowly stretch your leg until you feel stretching in the back side. Hold this for 4 long breaths before proceeding. Try to relax your back.

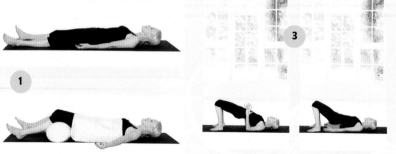

Lie on your back with your hands stretched out to the side or on your stomach. Close your eyes and let your body become heavy. Take 8 slow and deep breaths.

Hug your knees inwards toward your chest for a few breaths and then place your heels right under your knees and spread your toes. Press down the soles of your feet and the backside of your upper arms. Avoid tightening your buttocks too much. 4 breaths.

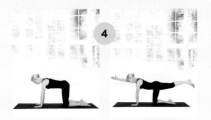

4

Come up to all fours and stretch your arms. Be sure to keep a straight line from your shoulder to your wrist and spread your fingers, keep the hip bones above your knees and push down the lower legs into the mat. Stretch out your right arm and left leg and then change sides. 4 breaths on each side.

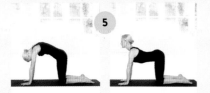

5

Strive to curve your spine and stretch out your thoracic spine and not the lumbar spine. 4 breaths.

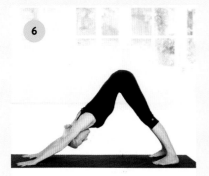

6

It is more important that the energy comes from your hands and that you stretch your spine than getting down with your heels into the mat. Reduce pressure in your shoulders by slightly bending your legs. 4 breaths.

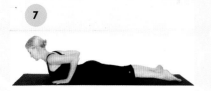

7

Press your legs and hands into the mat, and avoid tightening your buttocks too much here. Keep breathing calmly and deeply around the midriff. 4 breaths.

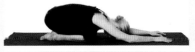

8

Extend your arms so that you experience a soft stretch in your shoulders. Breathe slowly and feel free to close your eyes. 8 breaths.

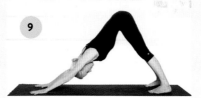

9

Now, you can "walk on the spot" in the Downward Dog Pose so that you bring some movement in to your legs. 4 breaths.

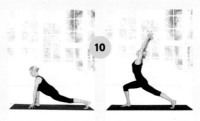

10

Inhale and lift your right leg, exhale and step forward with your foot between your hands. Stay for a few breaths and slowly get up with your upper body. Arms on your hips or up. Inhale and on exhalation get down to the Downward-Facing Dog Pose. Repeat on the left side.

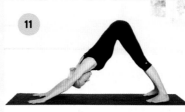

11

"Step on the spot" for movement in your legs. 4 breaths.

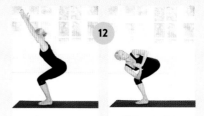

12

From the Downward-Facing Dog Pose, walk gently forward until you are standing upright on your feet. Exhale and bend your legs deeply, inhale and slowly lift your upper body and arms toward the ceiling. Modify by putting your hands on your hips, or advance by getting into a twist, first to one side and then to the other. Avoid adding weight on your toes, but let your hips move backward in order to feel your legs working. 4 breaths.

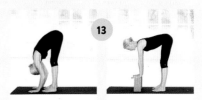

13

After a few breaths in the Chair Pose, exhale slowly and come into the Standing Forward Bend. Push off with your feet. Bend your knees if you feel stiff in your back or have trouble breathing. Simplify by putting your hands on blocks straight under your shoulders. Stay for 4 breaths.

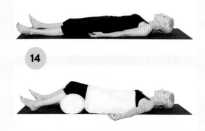

14

Come down on your back and take some well-earned breaths. Close your eyes and let your body become heavy. Take 20 slow and deep breaths (takes about 3 minutes).

Yin Yoga for Legs, Hips, and Lower Back

Start in the Butterfly Pose, where you'll stay for a minute and take long, deep breaths. Be deliberately very slow when you change poses (a bit like a sloth). Since yin yoga activates the connective tissue, which is a drier and tougher tissue than muscle tissue, it is especially important that the movements are extremely slow. This way, connective tissue is not contracted at once, which may hurt otherwise.

1. Butterfly Pose.
2. Wide-Angle Seated Forward Bend.
3. Head-to-Knee Pose, both sides.
4. All fours, Dragon Pose, both sides.
5. All fours, Cat/Cow Pose.
6. Child's Pose.
7. Corpse Pose.

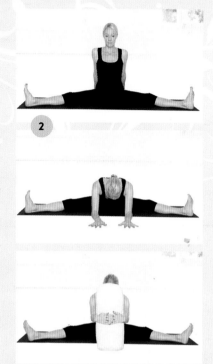

Stretch out your legs slowly to the side and relax your feet. Sit on a blanket or put blankets under your knees if discomfort occurs there. Stretch your back and get into a position where you feel a soft contact with the inside of your thighs. Stay and breathe slowly. Try to relax your legs and pelvis. 2 minutes.

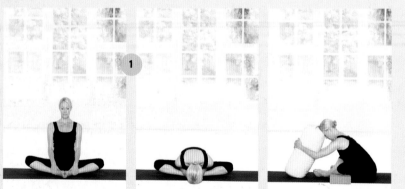

Sit with your feet together, perhaps on a folded blanket and with blocks under your thighs to prop up the hip. Stretch your lower back so that you do not slouch there. Breathe slowly. Close your eyes, listen to your breathing, and feel how the pelvis becomes heavy. Stay for 2 minutes.

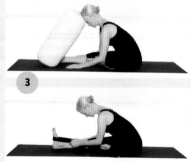

Slowly lead your left foot toward the right inside of your calf or thigh. You can put a blanket or a block under the bent leg for support. Gently stretch your lower back and then aim to fold your lower body forward slightly, just until you feel a gentle contact with the back of your thighs. 2 minutes. Repeat the movement on the other side.

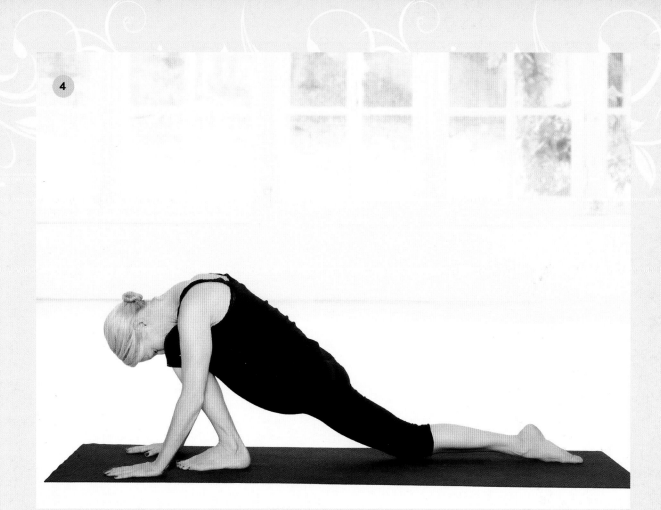

4

Gently move up to all fours. Stop and breathe a couple of times. Then step forward with your left foot and carefully lower your hips until you feel contact with the hip flexor, on the front of the left hip. Do not go fully out but stay where you make contact. Step gently back to all fours. 2 minutes. Repeat the movement on the other side.

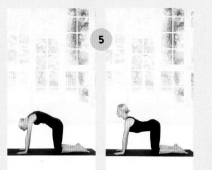

5

Try to curve your back and stretch it out into the thoracic spine and not the lumbar spine. 4 breaths.

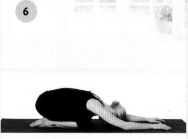

6

Extend your arms so that you experience a soft stretch in your shoulders. Take 4 slow breaths with your eyes closed.

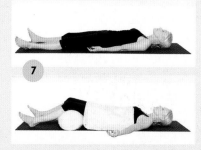

7

Come down on your back and take some well-earned breaths. Close your eyes and let your body become heavy. Take about 20 slow and deep breaths (usually takes around 3 minutes).

Strength and Energy

These exercises are done in one flow. When you are in a pose you inhale and any movement or deepening of the position occurs on exhalation. If the amount of time you should stay in the pose is not specified, it is more of a movement-based position, serving as a transition to the next pose.

1. Mountain Pose.
2. Standing Forward Bend.
3. Chair Pose, both sides.
4. Mountain Pose.
5. Crescent Moon Pose, right.
6. Mountain Pose.
7. Crescent Moon Pose, left.
8. Mountain Pose.
9. Warrior Pose 2, right leg.
10. Reverse Warrior Pose, right leg.
11. Warrior Pose 2, left leg.
12. Sun Warrior, left leg.
13. Wide-Legged Forward Bend.
14. Mountain Pose.
15. Swaying Palm Tree Pose, both sides.
16. Mountain Pose.
17. Rotated Chair Pose, both sides.
18. Standing Forward Bend.
19. Downward-Facing Dog Pose.
20. Half Pigeon Pose on your back, both sides.
21. Corpse Pose.

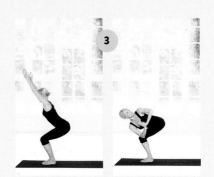

Exhale and bend deeply at the legs, inhale and slowly lift your upper body and arms toward the ceiling. Simplify by putting your hands on your hips, or advance by getting into a twist, first to one side and then to the other side. Avoid adding any weight at the front of your toes, but aim your hips backwards so that you feel your legs working. 4 breaths.

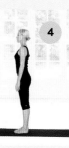

Push down the little toe, big toe, and the inside and outside of your heels until you feel that your legs become strong and active. Lengthen your spine and lift your chest. Fix your gaze straight ahead. Breathe through your diaphragm, taking 4 long, deep breaths.

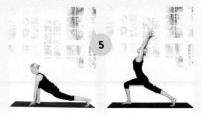

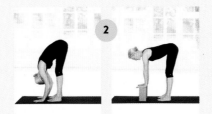

Inhale, step backwards with one leg. Hold for 2 breaths and step back to the Mountain Pose.

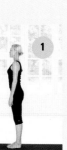

Push down your little toe, big toe, and the inside and outside of your heels until you feel that your legs become strong and active. Lengthen your spine and lift your chest. Fix your gaze straight ahead. Breathe through your diaphragm, taking 4 long, deep breaths.

Inhale in the Mountain Pose, bend your legs and exhale, and slowly fold your upper body down over your legs. Bend your knees if you feel stiffness in the back side or if you have trouble breathing freely. Simplify by placing your hands on blocks directly below your shoulders. Stay for 4 minutes.

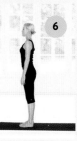

Push down the little toe, big toe, and the inside and outside of your heels until you feel that your legs have become strong and active. Lengthen your spine and lift your chest. Fix your gaze straight ahead. Breathe through your diaphragm, taking 4 long, deep breaths.

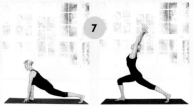

7

Inhale, step backwards with the other leg. Hold for two breaths and step back into the Mountain Pose.

8

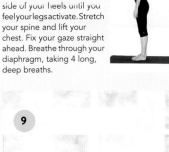

Push down your little toe, big toe, and the inside and outside of your heels until you feel your legs activate. Stretch your spine and lift your chest. Fix your gaze straight ahead. Breathe through your diaphragm, taking 4 long, deep breaths.

10

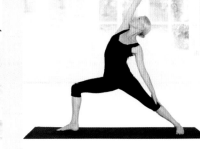

From Warrior Pose 2: Lift your right arm up until you feel a stretch on the right side, and lower your left hand and let it rest on the thigh behind. Hold for 2 breaths. Come back to Warrior Pose 2 and then to the Mountain Pose. 4 breaths.

9

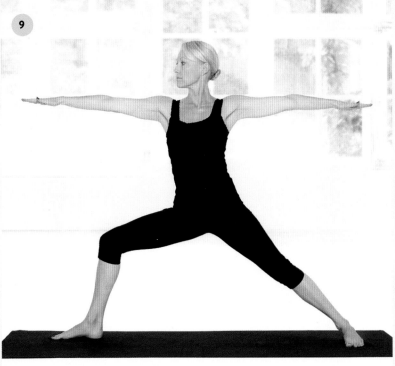

Take a step backward with your left leg and point the toes of your left foot outward from your hip. Stretch your rear leg. Hold for 2 breaths.

11

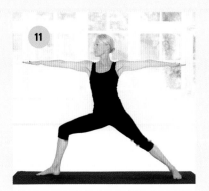

Now take a step backward with your right leg to Warrior Pose 2 and point the toes of your right foot outward from your hip. Stretch your rear leg. Hold for 2 breaths.

12

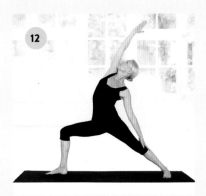

From Warrior Pose 2: Lift your left arm up until you feel a stretch on the left side, and lower your right hand and let it rest on your thigh. Hold for 2 breaths. Come back into the Warrior Pose B and then the Mountain Pose.

13

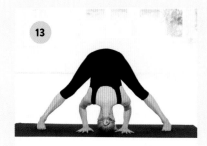

Take a big step to the side. Point your toes forward, keeping them parallel. Push your feet firmly down into the mat and gently fold your upper body forward over your legs. Hold for 4 breaths, then bend your knees and roll gently up and get into the Mountain Pose.

▶

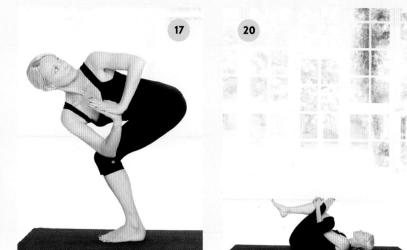

Push down the little toe, big toe, and the inside and outside of your heels until you feel that your legs have become strong and active. Lengthen your spine and lift your chest. Fix your gaze straight ahead. Breathe through your diaphragm, taking 4 long, deep breaths.

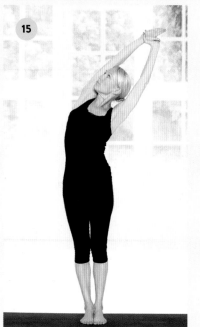

Inhale and bend slowly over to the right side until you feel a gentle stretch on your right side. Keep the power in your legs. Hold for 2 breaths and then come slowly back to the Mountain Pose, and then perform the Swaying Palm Tree Pose on your left side and hold for 2 breaths.

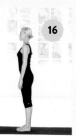

Push down the little toe, big toe, and the inside and outside of your heels until you feel that your legs have become strong and active. Lengthen your spine and lift your chest. Fix your gaze straight ahead. Breathe through your diaphragm, taking 4 long, deep breaths.

Exhale and bend deeply at the legs, inhale and slowly lift your upper body and arms toward the ceiling. Bring your arms together in front of your chest and get into a twist on your right side and place your left elbow on the outside of your right leg. 4 breaths. Repeat the same movement on your left side. Hold for 4 breaths.

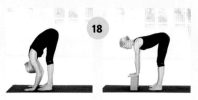

Exhale and slowly fold your upper body over your legs. Hold for 2 long breaths.

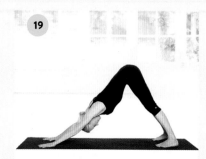

Put your hands down on the mat under your shoulders and step slowly backward with your feet to the Downward-Facing Dog Pose. Hold for 2 deep breaths.

Get slowly down on your back and put your feet on the mat under your knees. Put your left foot on your left thigh and lift your left leg. Insert your right hand between your legs and grab the lower leg and bring it toward you. Avoid lifting the lumbar spine and hip. Hold for 4 breaths. Change to your left side. Hold for 4 breaths.

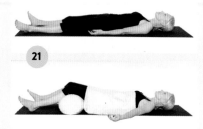

Stretch your legs out slowly until you are fully extended and take some well-earned breaths. Close your eyes and let your body get heavy. Take about 20 slow and deep breaths (usually takes around 3 minutes).

Yin Yoga for Chest and Lower Back

Here, you start with a gentle hip opener, the Butterfly Pose, to increase circulation in the spinal musculature with a twist. The Dragon Pose strengthens and creates greater elasticity in the hip flexors. This is followed by a soft chest and shoulder stretch or a twist to calm the body and mind. An excellent session to do after a day of sedentary work, for example.

1. Butterfly Pose.
2. Seated Twist, both sides.
3. Dragon Pose, both sides.
4. Chest and shoulder stretch or the Sewing Thread.
5. Child's Pose.
6. Corpse Pose.

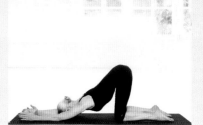

Move forward with your hands until you can lower your chest down toward the mat and keep a straight line from knee to hip. 2 minutes.

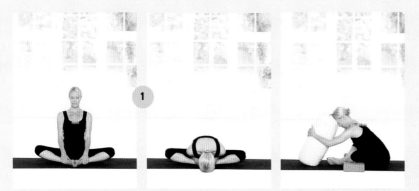

Sit with your feet together, perhaps on a folded blanket and with blocks under your thighs to prop up the hip. Stretch your lower back so you do not slouch down. Breathe slowly. Feel free to close your eyes and listen to your breathing, and feel how the pelvis becomes heavy. 2 minutes.

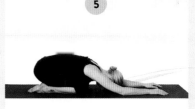

Get slowly back into the Child's Pose. Extend your knees to the side. Hold for 1 minute.

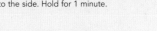

Slowly roll up to a sitting position with a stretched spine. Straighten your right leg and lift your left foot over your right leg. Hug your left knee with your right arm and gently stretch your back. Inhale and exhale, and turn smoothly over to the right. Focus your breathing to the left side of your chest. 2 minutes. Repeat the movement on the other side. Come slowly out of the position and in to the Child's Pose and take a few breaths.

Step slowly forward with your left foot and carefully lower your hips until you feel contact with the hip flexor in the front on your left hip. Do not go fully out but stay where you make contact. Step gently back to all fours. Repeat the movement on the other side. 2 minutes on each side.

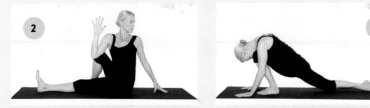

Get down on your back and take some well-earned breaths. Close your eyes and let your body become heavy. Take about 20 slow and deep breaths (usually takes about three minutes).

Balancing Sequence

Here is a session that works as much with activity as with recovery. You exercise stability and movement in the hip and spine with the Warrior exercises, and then increase the blood flow to the muscles in your neck and thoracic spine with the Dolphin, Cat/Cow, and Tiger Poses. The focus in this session is to synchronize the right and left side of the body and cerebral hemisphere with the help of alternating nostril breathing, and performing all the exercises on both right and left side. Strive to keep a steady pace of breathing such that inhalation is as long as exhalation on both sides.

1. The Accomplished Pose. *Nadi shodhana.*
2. On all fours, Tiger Pose.
3. Cat/Cow Pose.
4. Dolphin Pose.
5. Warrior Pose A, right.
6. Warrior Pose C, right.
7. Warrior Pose A, left.
8. Warrior Pose C, right.
9. Downward-Facing Dog Pose.
10. Lie on your back, Lying Spine Rotation.
11. Lie on a pillow, Legs Up Against the Wall.
12. Corpse Pose.

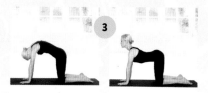

Try to curve your spine and stretch your thoracic spine and not the lumbar spine. 4 breaths.

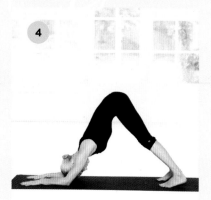

Position yourself on your forearms and push them down to the floor. Bring your chest forward and shoulders backward. Move backward with your feet and lift your buttocks toward the ceiling. If you feel too much stretching in the backside, bend your legs. Hold for 4 breaths and then come out of the position through the Downward-Facing Dog Pose.

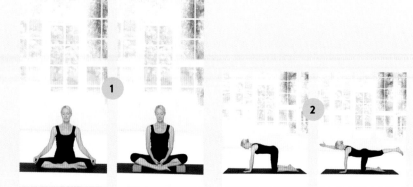

Try to sit up straight or against a wall. Inhale through one nostril and exhale through the other, inhale through the one you just exhaled through and exhale through the other. *Nadi shodhana,* 6 breaths. Then, tilt your head to the right until you feel a stretch on the side of your neck. Hold for 4 breaths and change slowly.

Get up on all fours and stretch your arms. Make sure you keep a straight line from your shoulders to your wrist, spread your fingers and keep the hip bones right over the knees and push down your lower legs into the mat. Stretch your right arm and left leg and then change sides. 4 breaths on each side.

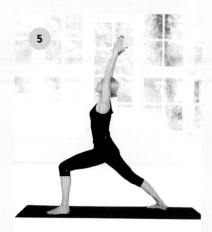

Here you step forward with your right foot and lower your left foot on the mat, inhale and come up with your upper body. Hold for 2 breaths.

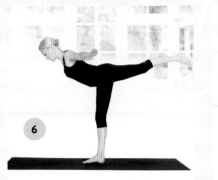

6

Put more emphasis on your right leg and lift your left leg off the mat. Hipbones pointing down and chest stretched forward. Get back to the Downward-Facing Dog Pose.

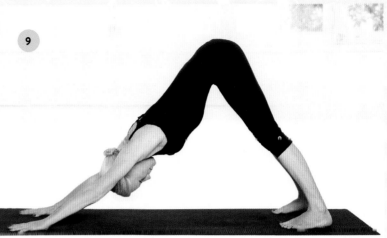

9

It is more important that the energy comes from your hands pressing down than to get your heels down into the mat. Reduce pressure in your shoulders by slightly bending your legs. Hold for 4 to 12 breaths.

7

Step forward with your left foot and lower your right foot on to the mat, inhale and come up with your upper body. Hold for 2 breaths.

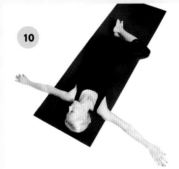

10

Get down on your back and hug your knees. Lower your feet on to the mat and extend your arms to the side. Fold both of your legs over to the right and then to the left. Hold for 4 breaths on each side.

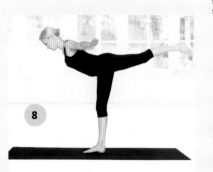

8

Put more emphasis on your left leg and lift your leg off the mat. Hip bones pointing down and chest stretched forward. Then get back to the Downward-Facing Dog Pose.

11

Lie straight and hug your knees. Put a blanket, pillow or a bolster under your lower back or stretch your legs toward the ceiling or up against a wall. Close your eyes and try to relax in your lower back for 8 long and deep breaths.

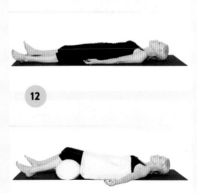

12

Slowly stretch out your legs until you are fully extended and take some well-earned breaths. Close your eyes and let your body become heavy. Take about 20 slow and deep breaths (usually takes around 3 minutes).

Soft Flow

In this session you want to move in pace with your breathing, so allow your breaths to be as slow and lengthy as possible, and perform movements while breathing. When you hold a pose, try to develop a sense of stability and lightness of body and mind through breathing, and note where in your body you feel contact while performing the movement. In the final meditation technique, you continue to work on trying to feel your body through your breath. Ask yourself these breathing questions: How does it feel? Where do you feel it? In what way does it feel? And try not to look for answers but let them come on their own. Here you exercise concentration and focus. Hold each pose for at least 4 long breaths.

1. Mountain Pose, breathe *ujjayi* 8 breaths.
2. Shoulder Stretch, 4 times forward and backward.
3. Cat/Cow Pose, 4 times and Tiger Pose. Hold each side for 4 breaths each. Cobra Pose. (Or two Sun Salutations if you are familiar with the sequence).
4. Downward-Facing Dog Pose.
5. Crescent Moon Pose, both sides.
6. Downward-Facing Dog Pose.
7. Half Pigeon on your back, both sides.
8. Child's Pose.
9. Full Forward Bend.
10. Lying Back Rotation, both sides.
11. Corpse Pose.
12. Seated. *Apa japa.*

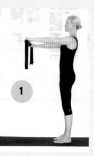

Push down your little and big toe, and the inside and outside of your heels until you feel pressure in your legs. Stretch your spine and lift your chest. Fix your gaze straight ahead. Breathe through your diaphragm and take long, deep breaths with more sound in the breath. 8 breaths.

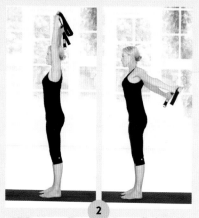

Inhale and roll your shoulders forward and upward, exhale and roll your shoulders back and downward 4 times, then switch sides.

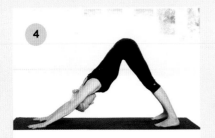

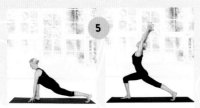

Perform the Cat/Cow Pose 4 times and then the Tiger Pose 4 times. Hold each side for 4 breaths. Follow with your breath in the movements. (You can also do two Sun Salutations if you are familiar with the sequence.)

4

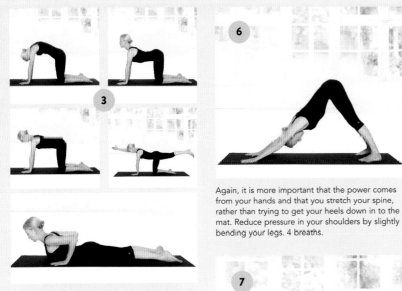

It is important that the power comes from your hands and that you stretch your spine, than to get your heels down in to the mat. Reduce pressure in your shoulders by slightly bending your legs. 4 breaths.

5

From the Downward-Facing Dog Pose, inhale, lift your right leg, and take a step forward with your right foot. Hold for 2 breaths and step back into the Downward-Facing Dog Pose. Repeat the same thing on the left side.

6

Again, it is more important that the power comes from your hands and that you stretch your spine, rather than trying to get your heels down in to the mat. Reduce pressure in your shoulders by slightly bending your legs. 4 breaths.

7

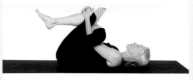

Get slowly down on your back and press your feet in to the mat under your knees. Put your left foot on your right thigh, and lift your left leg. Insert your left hand between your legs and grab your lower leg and move it toward you. Avoid lifting the lumbar spine and hip. Hold for 4 breaths. Change sides slowly and repeat the movement.

8

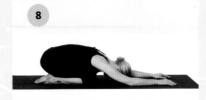

Get up on all fours, put your knees down on the floor, and rest your stomach on your thighs. Slowly stretch your arms forward. Hold for 4 breaths.

9

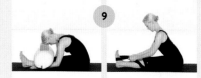

Get up to a sitting position and stretch your legs. Strive to have activity in your legs and stretch your back. Fold your upper body forward and try to have a straight back.

10

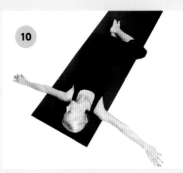

Slowly get down on your back and hug your knees. Lower your feet onto the mat and extend your arms. Fold your legs over to one side and turn your head and look over your arm on the opposite side so that you get a twist in your back. Then change sides on each leg and *drishti*. Hold for 4 breaths on each side.

11

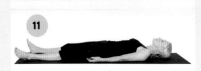

Lie on your back and stretch out your legs slowly until you are fully extended, and take a few well-earned breaths. Close your eyes and let your body become heavy. Take around 15 slow and deep breaths (takes around 2 minutes).

12

Come slowly over to the right and then up to a sitting position. Sit comfortably and close your eyes. Stay like this for a few minutes and just observe your breath. If you have more time, stay for 10 to 15 minutes.

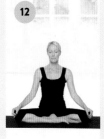

Restore Energy and Meditative Focus

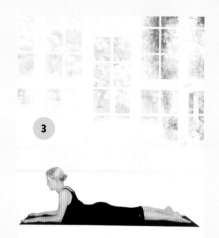

Here you get to exercise your breath and let go of stress in your body and mind. Play some nice music, light a candle, and dim the lights. Feel free to keep your eyes closed while performing your yoga. Allow your breath to be slow, soft, and deep. If you lose concentration, focus again on your breathing.

1. Child's Pose.
2. Half Pigeon Pose, both sides.
3. Sphinx/Seal Pose.
4. Half Spinal Twist, both sides.
5. Lie on a pillow with your legs up against a wall.
6. Corpse Pose.
7. The Accomplished Pose, breathing *apa japa*.

Get down on your stomach, lie on your forearms and to begin, rest your stomach on the mat. Relax your buttocks and legs. 2 minutes. Get back into the Child's Pose.

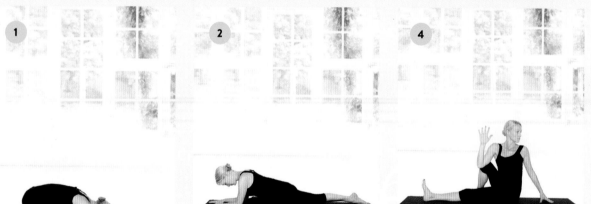

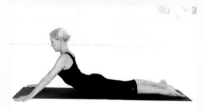

Sit on your knees and rest your stomach on your thighs, stretch your arms forward and rest your forehead on the floor. Extend your knees to the side if it feels better for your back. Relax your shoulders and arms. 1 minute.

From all fours, bring your right knee toward your right hand and fold in your lower leg diagonally across the mat below you. Lower your hips until you feel a contact with the outside of your buttocks or hips. 1 minute. Come slowly back to all fours and change legs at a slow pace.

Come slowly up to a sitting position with your spine stretched. Straighten your right leg and lift your left foot over your right leg. Hug your left knee with your right arm and gently stretch your back. Inhale and exhale and gently twist your upper body to the left. Focus your breathing to the left side of your chest. 1 minute. Slowly change sides and repeat the movement.

5

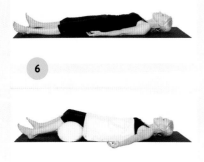

Slowly come down on your back and hug your knees. Put a blanket, pillow, or a bolster under your lower back or stretch your legs up toward the ceiling or up against a wall. Lie here and close your eyes and try to relax in your lower back during 8 long and deep breaths, or around 2 minutes.

6

Stretch out your legs slowly until you are fully extended and take a few well-earned breaths. Close your eyes and let your body become heavy. Take about 20 slow and deep breaths (usually takes around 3 minutes).

7

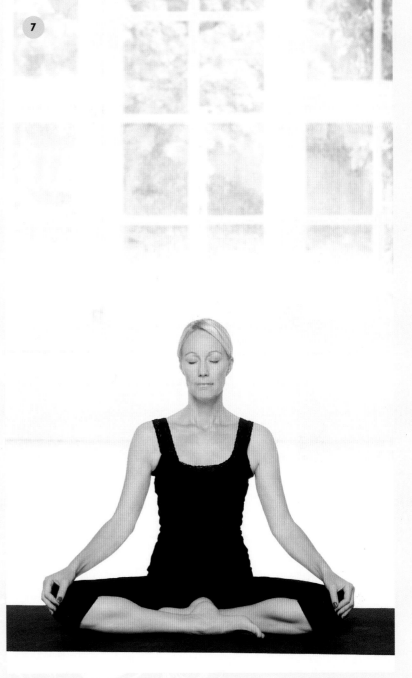

Come slowly over to your right side and then up to a sitting position. Sit down comfortably and close your eyes. Breathe *apa japa* for 3 minutes. Stay for another couple of minutes and just observe your breath. If you have more time, stay for 10–15 minutes.

INDEX

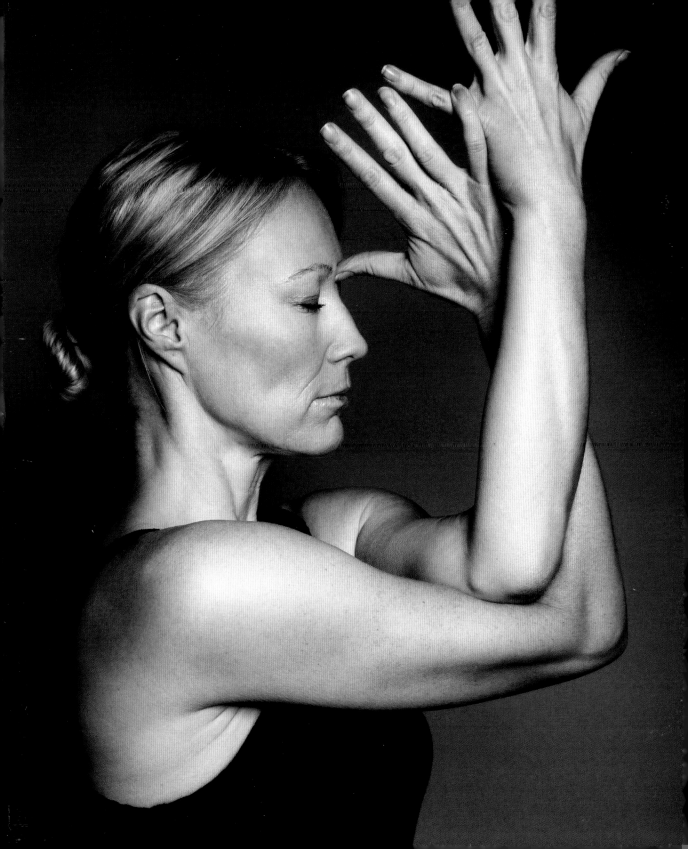

ACKNOWLEDGMENTS

I want to express my gratitude to my dear sister, Lotta, who has stood by my side all my life, through thick and thin. We share the interest for health and yoga, and we are both passionate about life. THANK YOU for being in my life, for giving me love and support.

Magnus, without you I would not have been able to do this. You are there all the time as my stable oak. You create space for me. You take as much responsibility for our family as I do. And you never doubt me. You challenge me with love to grow as a person. You are my best friend, husband, and the father of my children.

Thank you Mom! When I think of everything you have given me, I become speechless. And I feel so much love and gratitude toward you. You are the most generous and genuinely good person I know. You are one of my primary role models in life.

Alan. My mentor, yoga master, and friend. You have helped me to regain faith in myself and in what I can do. You inspired me to let go of what I held onto and what did not allow me to get any stronger. For that, I will be eternally grateful to you. You see me. And I appreciate your sincerity, your life history, your ability to be yourself, your way of guiding and showing us, your students, the strength to evolve to become our best without sacrificing ourselves on the way. You have helped me bring forth the inner grace in myself, the one who not only is but does. By working with you I found my way back to the child in me. And I finally found the strength to let go of the mantel I have been carrying around for so long. THANK YOU.

Thanks to all my students, colleagues, and amazing friends for all the support during this writing process. Without you, I would not have been where I am.

Andreas, you did it again. Thank you.

Thank you to Bonnier Fakta and Kerstin Bergfors, and extra thank you to you Alexandra Lindén and Anders Timrén for your fine work and dedication. It has been a true pleasure to work with you.